KETO DIET

COOKBOOK FOR BEGINNERS 250 RECIPES

A Simple Cookbook To Achieve Weight Loss, Boost Your Energy, and Reboot Your Metabolism With Tasty Recipes

Table of Contents

Introduction

For the benefits of weight loss, the ketogenic diet has been widely commended and praised. It has been shown that this high-fat, low-carb diet is highly balanced overall. It really makes your body, like a talking machine, burn fat. It is also respected by public figures. But the question is, how can ketosis increase the loss of weight? The following is a comprehensive picture of the process of ketosis and weight loss.

Ketosis is considered rare by some people. Even though several nutritionists and physicians have approved it. It is still disapproved of by many people. The misconceptions are attributable to the myths about the ketogenic diet that have spread.

When the body is out of glucose, it relies on stored fat immediately. It is also important to note that glucose is created by carbohydrates and you will also be able to lower your glucose levels once you begin a low carbohydrate diet. Then, instead of carbohydrates, that is, glucose, your body can generate fuel by fat.

The mechanism of accumulating fat via fat is known as ketosis, and it becomes extremely effective at burning excess fat once your body enters this state. Also, as during the ketogenic diet, glucose levels are low, the body gains many other health benefits.

A ketogenic diet is not only good for weight loss, it also helps in a positive way to boost your overall health. Ketogenic focuses on placing the body in a natural metabolic state, that is, ketosis, unlike all other diet plans, which focus on decreasing calorie intake. The only thing that makes this diet controversial is that it is not very well thought out for this kind of metabolism. Your body will easily burn accumulated fat by having tattoos on your body regularly, leading to great weight loss.

The query arises now. How does the human body become affected by ketosis?

This process does not last more than 2-3 days, however. This is the time the human body takes to reach the process of ketosis. You are not going to have any side effects until you get in.

You should also begin reducing the consumption of calories and carbohydrates gradually. The most common mistake dietitians make is that, at the same time, they want to begin removing something from their diet. This is where the issue occurs. When you restrict all at once, the human body can respond extremely negatively. You've got to begin gradually. Read this guide to learn more about how the ketogenic diet can be treated after 50.

Most fats are healthy and important to our health, so essential fatty acids and essential amino acids are available (proteins). The most powerful source of energy is fat, and every gram contains around 9 calories. This more than doubles the sum of protein and carbohydrates (both have 4 calories per gram).

Your body adjusts and converts the fat and protein, as well as the fat it has accumulated, into ketones or ketones for energy when you consume a lot of fat and protein and substantially reduce carbohydrates. This mechanism of metabolism is called ketosis. The ketogen in the ketogenic diet comes from here.

CHAPTER 1:

Breakfast

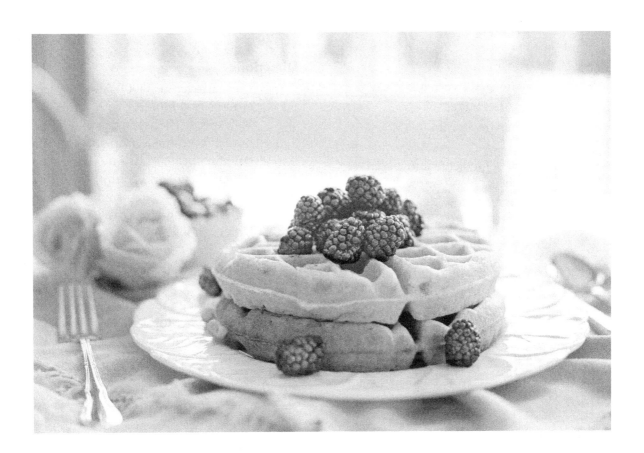

Almond Flour Pancakes

Preparation Time: 5 minutes
Cooking Time: 5 minutes
Servings: 4
Ingredients

- ½ cup almond flour
- ½ cup cream cheese
- 4 medium eggs
- ½ tsp cinnamon
- ½ tsp granulated sweetener
- 1 tsp grass-fed butter
- 1 tbsp sugar-free syrup

Directions

1. Add all the ingredients into a blender and let them blend in well. Once done, set the batter aside.
2. On a non-stick pan at medium heat, fry pancakes with melted butter. Once the center starts to bubble, turn over. Once done with the pancake, move on to the rest, using the batter.
3. Finally, serve your pancakes warm, along with some low carb fruit or with an exquisite side of sugar-free syrup to enjoy a healthy and tasty breakfast.

Nutrition:
Calories: 234
Fat: 20g
Carbohydrates: 4g
Fiber: 1.5g
Net carbs: 2.5g
Protein: 11g

Avocado Toast

Preparation Time: 20 minutes
Cooking Time: 40 minutes
Servings: 2

Ingredients

- ½ cup grass-fed butter
- 2 tbsp coconut oil
- 7 large eggs
- 1 tsp baking powder
- 2 cups almond flour
- ½ tsp xanthan gum
- ½ tsp kosher salt
- 1 medium avocado

Directions

1. Preheat over at 3500F. Beat eggs for around two minutes with a mixer at high speed. Then, add coconut oil and butter (both melted) to the eggs and continue beating. Ensure that oil and butter are not too warm to cook the eggs. Add remaining bread ingredients and mix well. Now, the batter should become thick. Pour batter in a non-stick loaf pan lined with parchment paper. Let it bake for 45 minutes or until the fork comes clean through the middle.
2. For topping, toast two slices of your keto bread to your liking. Slice the whole avocado thinly, without the skin or pit. Use these to make one long strip of overlapping slices. Roll these into a spiral and that is it! Enjoy your keto bread with avocado topping.

Nutrition:
Calories: 350
Fat: 32g
Carbohydrates: 7g
Fiber: 4g
Net carbs: 3g
Protein: 10g

Chicken Avocado Egg Bacon Salad

Preparation Time: 10 minutes

Cooking Time: 10 minutes

Servings: 4

Ingredients

- 12 oz. cooked chicken breast
- 6 slices crumbled bacon
- 3 boiled eggs cut into cubes
- 1 cup cherry tomatoes cut into halves
- 1/2 small sliced red onion
- 1 large avocado(s)
- 1/2 stick finely chopped celery
- Salad Dressing
- 1/2 cup olive oil mayonnaise
- 2 tbsp. sour cream
- 1 tsp Dijon mustard
- 4 tbsp. extra virgin olive oil
- 2 cloves minced garlic
- 2 tsp lemon juice
- 4 cups lettuce
- Salt and pepper to taste

Directions

1. Combine all the ingredients together and mix them well for the salad dressing. Then, combine chicken, tomatoes, bacon, eggs, red onions, and celery together. Add about ¾ of the salad dressing and mix them well. Add the avocado and toss together gently. Check the taste and, if needed, add the remainder of the salad dressing as well. Finally, add salt and pepper to taste and then serve it over lettuce.

Nutrition:

Calories: 387 Fat: 27g Carbohydrates: 2.5g

Fiber: 1g Net carbs: 1.5g

Protein: 24g

Bacon Wrapped Chicken Breast

Preparation Time: 10 minutes

Cooking Time: 45 minutes

Servings: 4

Ingredients

- 4 boneless, skinless chicken breast
- 8 oz. sharp cheddar cheese
- 8 slices bacon
- 4 oz. sliced jalapeno peppers
- 1 tsp garlic powder
- Salt and pepper to taste

Directions

1. Preheat the oven at around 3500F. Ensure to season both sides of chicken breast well with salt, garlic powder, and pepper. Place the chicken breast on a non-stick baking sheet (foil-covered). Cover the chicken with cheese and add jalapeno slices. Cut the bacon slices in half and then place the four halves over each piece of chicken. Bake for around 30 to 45 minutes at most. If the chicken is set but the bacon still feels undercooked, you may want to put it under the broiler for a few minutes. Once done, serve hot with a side of low carb garlic parmesan roasted asparagus.

Nutrition:

Calories: 640

Fat: 48g

Carbohydrates: 6g

Fiber: 3g

Net carbs: 3g

Protein: 47g

Egg Salad

Preparation Time: 15 minutes

Cooking Time: 10 minutes

Servings: 4

Ingredients

- 6 eggs
- 2 tbsp mayonnaise
- 1 tsp Dijon mustard
- 1 tsp lemon juice
- Salt and pepper to taste

Directions

1. In a medium saucepan, place the solid eggs gently.
2. Add some cold water so that the eggs are covered around an inch. Boil them for around 10 minutes.
3. Once done, remove them from the heat and let them cool. Peel the eggs while running them under cold water. Now add these in a food processor and pulse until they are chopped.
4. Add and stir mayonnaise, lemon juice, mustard, and salt and pepper. Ensure to taste and then adjust as necessary.
5. Finally, serve them with a bit of lettuce leaves and, if needed, bacon for wrapping.

Nutrition:

Calories: 222 Fat: 19g

Net carbs: 1g

Protein: 13g

Blueberry Muffins

Preparation Time: 10 minutes

Cooking Time: 30 minutes

Servings: 12

Ingredients

- 1 container Greek yogurt

- 3 large eggs
- 1/2 tsp vanilla extract
- 1/4 tsp salt
- 2 1/2 cups almond flour
- 1/4 cup Swerve sweetener (add more if using plain Greek yogurt)
- 2 tsp baking powder
- Water if needed to thin
- 1/2 cup fresh blueberries

Directions

1. Preheat oven at 325°F. Simultaneously, line-up a clean muffin pan with around 12 parchment liners. Combine yogurt, vanilla, eggs, and salt in a blender. Blend the mixture till it is smooth. Add almond flour, baking powder and sweetener. Now, blend again until it is smooth. If the batter is thick, add one tablespoon of water at a time. The batter should be thick, but it must be pourable.
2. Add in blueberries and divide these equally for the prepared muffin cups. Finally, bake these for 25 to 30 minutes. Use a tester and insert it right in the middle. If it comes out clean, your muffins are ready.

Nutrition:

Calories: 163 Net carbs: 3.8g

Fat: 12.9g

Protein: 7.6g

Bacon Hash

Preparation Time: 5 minutes

Cooking Time: 10 minutes

Servings: 2

Ingredients:

- Small green pepper (1)

- Jalapenos (2)
- Small onion (1)
- Eggs (4)
- Bacon slices (6)

Directions:

1. Chop the bacon into chunks using a food processor. Set aside for now. Slice the onions and peppers into thin strips. Dice the jalapenos as small as possible.
2. Heat a skillet and fry the veggies. Once browned, combine the fixings and cook until crispy. Place on a serving dish with the eggs.

Nutrition:

Carbohydrates: 9 grams

Protein: 23 grams

Fats: 24 grams

Calories: 366

Bagels with Cheese

Preparation Time: 10 minutes

Cooking Time: 15 minutes

Servings: 6

Ingredients:

- Mozzarella cheese (2.5 cups)
- Baking powder (1 tsp.)
- Cream cheese (3 oz.)
- Almond flour (1.5 cups)
- Eggs (2)

Directions:

1. Shred the mozzarella and combine with the flour, baking powder, and cream cheese in a mixing container. Pop into the microwave for about one minute. Mix well.
2. Let the mixture cool and add the eggs. Break apart into six sections and shape into round bagels. Note: You can also sprinkle with a seasoning of your choice or pinch of salt if desired.
3. Bake them for approximately 12 to 15 minutes. Serve or cool and store.

Nutrition:

Carbohydrates: 8 grams

Protein: 19 grams Fats: 31 grams

Calories: 374

Cauli Flitters

Preparation Time: 10 minutes

Cooking Time: 15 minutes

Servings: 2

Ingredients:

- 2 eggs
- 1 head of cauliflower
- 1 tbsp. yeast
- sea salt, black pepper
- 1-2 tbsp. ghee
- 1 tbsp. turmeric
- 2/3 cup almond flour

Directions:

1. Place the cauliflower into a large pot and start to boil it for 8 mins. Add the florets into a food processor and pulse them.
2. Add the eggs, almond flour, yeast, turmeric, salt and pepper to a mixing bowl. Stir well. Form into patties.
3. Heat your ghee to medium in a skillet. Form your fritters and cook until golden on each side (3-4 mins).
4. Serve it while hot.

Nutrition:

Calories: 238 kcal Fat: 23 g

Carbs: 5 g Protein: 6 g

Scrambled Eggs

Preparation Time: 2 minutes

Cooking Time: 8 minutes

Servings: 4

Ingredients:

- 4 oz. butter
- 8 eggs
- salt and pepper for taste

Directions:

1. Crack the eggs in a bowl, and whisk them together, while seasoning it.
2. Melt the butter in a skillet over medium heat, but don't turn it into brown.
3. Pour the eggs into the skillet and cook it for 1-2 mins, until they look and feel fluffy and creamy.
4. Tip: If you want to shake things up, you can pair this one up with bacon, salmon, or maybe avocado as well.

Nutrition:

Carbs: 1 g Fat: 31 g

Protein: 11 g

Calories: 327 kcal

Frittata with Spinach

Preparation Time: 5 minutes

Cooking Time: 30 minutes

Servings: 4

Ingredients:

- 8 eggs
- 8 ozs. fresh spinach
- 5 ozs. diced bacon
- 5 ozs. shredded cheese
- 1 cup heavy whipping cream
- 2 tbsps. butter
- salt and pepper

Directions:

1. Preheat the oven to 350 °F
2. Fry the bacon until crispy, add the spinach and cook until wilted. Set them aside.
3. Whisk the cream and eggs together, and pour it into the baking dish.
4. Add the cheese, spinach, and bacon on the top, and place in the oven. Bake for 25-30 minutes, until golden brown on top.

Nutrition:

Carbs: 4 g

Fat: 59 g

Protein: 27 g

Calories: 661 kcal

Cheese Omelet

Preparation Time: 5 minutes

Cooking Time: 10 minutes

Servings: 2

Ingredients:

- 6 eggs
- 3 ozs. ghee
- 7 ozs. shredded cheddar cheese
- salt and pepper

Directions:

1. Whisk the eggs until smooth. Compound half of the cheese and season it with salt and pepper.
2. Melt the butter in a pan. Pour in the mixture and let it sit for a few minutes (3-4)
3. When the mixture is looking good, add the other half of the cheese. Serve immediately.

Nutrition:

Carbs: 4 g Fat: 80 g Protein: 40 g

Calories: 897 kcal

Capicola Egg Cups

Preparation Time: 5 minutes

Cooking Time: 15 minutes

Servings: 4

Ingredients:

- 8 eggs
- 1 cup cheddar cheese
- 4 oz. capicola or bacon (slices)
- salt, pepper, basil

Directions:

1. Preheat the oven to 400°F. You will need 8 wells of a standard-size muffin pan.
2. Place the slices in the 8 wells, forming a cup shape. Sprinkle into each cup some of the cheese, according to your liking.
3. Crack an egg into each cup, season them with salt and pepper.
4. Bake for 10-15 mins. Serve hot, top it with basil.

Nutrition:

Carbs: 1 g Fat: 11 g

Protein: 16 g

Calories: 171 kcal

Overnight "noats"

Preparation Time: 5 minutes plus overnight to chill

Cooking Time: 10 minutes

Servings: 1

Ingredients:

- 2 tablespoons hulled hemp seeds
- 1 tablespoon chia seeds
- ½ scoop (about 8 grams) collagen powder
- ½ cup unsweetened nut or seed milk (hemp, almond, coconut, and cashew)

Direction:

1. In a small mason jar or glass container, combine the hemp seeds, chia seeds, collagen, and milk.
2. Secure tightly with a lid, shake well, and refrigerate overnight.

Nutrition:

Calories: 263

Total Fat: 19g Protein: 16g

Total Carbs: 7g

Fiber: 5g

Net Carbs: 2g

Frozen keto coffee

Preparation Time: 5 minutes

Cooking Time: 20 minutes

Servings: 1

Ingredients:

- 12 ounces coffee, chilled
- 1 scoop MCT powder (or 1 tablespoon MCT oil)
- 1 tablespoon heavy (whipping) cream
- Pinch ground cinnamon
- Dash sweetener (optional)
- ½ cup ice

Directions:

1. In a blender, combine the coffee, MCT powder, cream, cinnamon, sweetener (if using), and ice. Blend until smooth.

Nutrition:

Calories: 127;

Total Fat: 13g;

Protein: 1g; Total Carbs: 1.5g;

Fiber: 1g;

Net Carbs: 0.5g

Easy Skillet Pancakes

Preparation Time: 5 minutes

Cooking Time: 5 minutes

Servings: 8

Ingredients:

- 8 ounces cream cheese
- 8 eggs
- 2 tablespoons coconut flour
- 2 teaspoons baking powder
- 1 teaspoon ground cinnamon
- ½ teaspoon vanilla extract
- 1 teaspoon liquid stevia or sweetener of choice (optional)
- 2 tablespoons butter

Directions

1. In a blender, combine the cream cheese, eggs, coconut flour, baking powder, cinnamon, vanilla, and stevia (if using). Blend until smooth.
2. In a large skillet over medium heat, melt the butter.
3. Use half the mixture to pour four evenly sized pancakes and cook for about a minute, until you see bubbles on top. Flip the pancakes and cook for another minute. Remove from the pan and add more butter or oil to the skillet if needed. Repeat with the remaining batter.
4. Top with butter and eat right away, or freeze the pancakes in a freezer-safe resealable bag with sheets of parchment in between, for up to 1 month.

Nutrition:

Calories: 179 Total Fat: 15g

Protein: 8g Total Carbs: 3g

Fiber: 1g Net Carbs: 2g

Quick Keto Blender Muffins

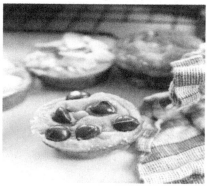

Preparation Time: 5 minutes

Cooking Time: 25 minutes

Servings: 12

Ingredients

- Butter, ghee, or coconut oil for greasing the pan
- 6 eggs
- 8 ounces cream cheese, at room temperature
- 2 scoops flavored collagen powder
- 1 teaspoon ground cinnamon
- 1 teaspoon baking powder
- Few drops or dash sweetener (optional)

Directions:

1. Preheat the oven to 350°F. Grease a 12-cup muffin pan very well with butter, ghee, or coconut oil. Alternatively, you can use silicone cups or paper muffin liners.
2. In a blender, combine the eggs, cream cheese, collagen powder, cinnamon, baking powder, and sweetener (if using). Blend until well combined and pour the mixture into the muffin cups, dividing equally.
3. Bake for 22 to 25 minutes until the muffins are golden brown on top and firm.

4. Let cool then store in a glass container or plastic bag in the refrigerator for up to 2 weeks or in the freezer for up to 3 months.

5. To Servings refrigerated muffins, heat in the microwave for 30 seconds. To Servings from frozen, thaw in the refrigerator overnight and then microwave for 30 seconds, or microwave straight from the freezer for 45 to 60 seconds or until heated through.

Nutrition:

Calories: 120 Total Fat: 10g

Protein: 6g Total Carbs: 1.5g

Fiber: 0g

Net Carbs: 1.5g

Keto Everything Bagels

Preparation Time: 10 minutes

Cooking Time: 15 minutes

Servings: 8

Ingredients:

- 2 cups shredded mozzarella cheese
- 2 tablespoons labneh cheese (or cream cheese)
- 1½ cups almond flour
- 1 egg
- 2 teaspoons baking powder
- ¼ teaspoon sea salt
- 1 tablespoon

Directions

1. Preheat the oven to 400°F.
2. In a microwave-safe bowl, combine the mozzarella and labneh cheeses. Microwave for 30 seconds, stir, then microwave for another 30 seconds. Stir well. If not melted completely,

microwave for another 10 to 20 seconds.

3. Add the almond flour, egg, baking powder, and salt to the bowl and mix well. Form into a dough using a spatula or your hands.

4. Cut the dough into 8 roughly equal pieces and form into balls.

5. Roll each dough ball into a cylinder, then pinch the ends together to seal.

6. Place the dough rings in a nonstick donut pan or arrange them on a parchment paper–lined baking sheet.

7. Sprinkle with the seasoning and bake for 12 to 15 minutes or until golden brown.

8. Store in plastic bags in the freezer and defrost overnight in the refrigerator. Reheat in the oven or toaster for a quick grab-and-go breakfast.

Nutrition:

Calories: 241

Total Fat: 19g

Protein: 12g

Total Carbs: 5.5g

Fiber: 2.5g

Net Carbs: 3g

Turmeric Chicken and Kale Salad with Food, Lemon and Honey

Preparation Time: 20 minutes

Cooking Time: 15 minutes

Servings: 4

Ingredients:

- For the chicken:
- 1 teaspoon of clarified butter or 1 tablespoon of coconut oil
- ½ medium brown onion, diced

- 250-300 g / 9 ounces minced chicken meat or diced chicken legs
- 1 large garlic clove, diced
- 1 teaspoon of turmeric powder
- 1 teaspoon of lime zest
- ½ lime juice
- ½ teaspoon of salt + pepper
- For the salad:
- 6 stalks of broccoli or 2 cups of broccoli flowers
- 2 tablespoons of pumpkin seeds (seeds)
- 3 large cabbage leaves, stems removed and chopped
- ½ sliced avocado
- Handful of fresh coriander leaves, chopped
- Handful of fresh parsley leaves, chopped
- For the dressing:
- 3 tablespoons of lime juice
- 1 small garlic clove, diced or grated
- 3 tablespoons of virgin olive oil (I used 1 tablespoon of avocado oil and 2 tablespoons of EVO)
- 1 teaspoon of raw honey
- ½ teaspoon whole or Dijon mustard
- ½ teaspoon of sea salt with pepper

Directions:

1. Heat the coconut oil in a pan. Add the onion and sauté over medium heat for 4-5 minutes, until golden brown. Add the minced chicken and garlic and stir 2-3 minutes over medium-high heat, separating.
2. Add your turmeric, lime zest, lime juice, salt and pepper, and cook, stirring consistently, for another 3-4 minutes. Set the ground beef aside.

3. While your chicken is cooking, put a small saucepan of water to the boil. Add your broccoli and cook for 2 minutes. Rinse with cold water and cut into 3-4 pieces each.
4. Add the pumpkin seeds to the chicken pan and toast over medium heat for 2 minutes, frequently stirring to avoid burning. Season with a little salt. Set aside. Raw pumpkin seeds are also good to use.
5. Put the chopped cabbage in a salad bowl and pour it over the dressing. Using your hands, mix, and massage the cabbage with the dressing. This will soften the cabbage, a bit like citrus juice with fish or beef Carpaccio: it "cooks" it a little.
6. Finally, mix the cooked chicken, broccoli, fresh herbs, pumpkin seeds, and avocado slices.

Nutrition:

232 calories

Fat 11

Fiber 9

Carbs 8

Protein 14

Buckwheat Spaghetti with Chicken Cabbage and Savory Food Recipes in Mass Sauce

Preparation Time: 15 minutes

Cooking Time: 15 minutes'

Servings: 2

Ingredients:

- For the noodles:
- 2-3 handfuls of cabbage leaves (removed from the stem and cut)

- Buckwheat noodles 150g / 5oz (100% buckwheat, without wheat)
- 3-4 shiitake mushrooms, sliced
- 1 teaspoon of coconut oil or butter
- 1 brown onion, finely chopped
- 1 medium chicken breast, sliced or diced
- 1 long red pepper, thinly sliced (seeds in or out depending on how hot you like it)
- 2 large garlic cloves, diced
- 2-3 tablespoons of Tamari sauce (gluten-free soy sauce)
- For the miso dressing:
- 1 tablespoon and a half of fresh organic miso
- 1 tablespoon of Tamari sauce
- 1 tablespoon of extra virgin olive oil
- 1 tablespoon of lemon or lime juice
- 1 teaspoon of sesame oil (optional)

Directions:

1. Boil a medium saucepan of water. Add the black cabbage and cook 1 minute, until it is wilted. Remove and reserve, but reserve the water and return to boiling. Add your soba noodles and cook according to the directions on the package (usually about 5 minutes). Rinse with cold water and reserve.

2. In the meantime, fry the shiitake mushrooms in a little butter or coconut oil (about a teaspoon) for 2-3 minutes, until its color is lightly browned on each side. Sprinkle with sea salt and reserve.

3. In that same pan, heat more coconut oil or lard over medium-high heat. Fry the onion and chili for 2-3 minutes, and then add the chicken pieces. Cook 5 minutes on medium heat, stirring a few times, then add the garlic, tamari sauce, and a little water. Cook for another 2-3 minutes, stirring continuously until your chicken is cooked.

4. Finally, add the cabbage and soba noodles and stir the chicken to warm it.

5. Stir the miso sauce and sprinkle the noodles at the end of the cooking, in this way you will keep alive all the beneficial probiotics in the miso.

Nutrition:

305 calories

Fat 11

Fiber 7

Carbs 9

Protein 12

CHAPTER 2:

Lunch

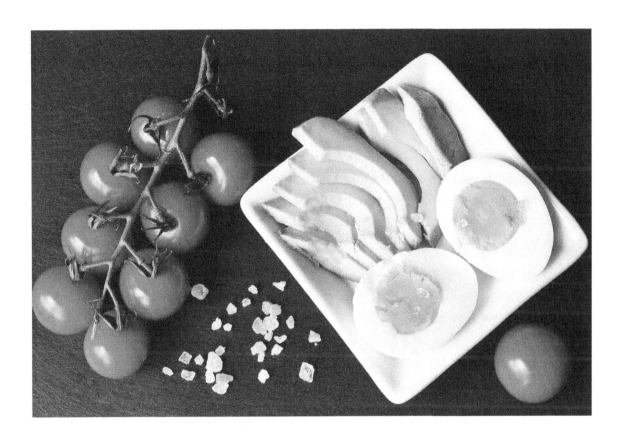

Chicken in Sweet and Sour Sauce with Corn Salad

Preparation Time: 10 minutes

Cooking Time: 15 minutes

Servings: 4

Ingredients:

- 2 cups plus 2 tablespoons of unflavored low-fat yoghurt
- 2 cups of frozen mango chunks
- 3 tablespoons of honey
- ¼ cup plus 1 tablespoon apple cider vinegar
- ¼ cup sultana
- 2 tablespoons of olive oil, plus an amount to be brushed
- ¼ teaspoon of cayenne pepper
- 5 dried tomatoes (not in oil)
- 2 small cloves of garlic, finely chopped
- 4 cobs, peeled
- 8 peeled and boned chicken legs, peeled (about 700g)
- Halls
- 6 cups of mixed salad
- 2 medium carrots, finely sliced

Directions:

1. For the smoothie: in a blender, mix 2 cups of yogurt, 2 cups of ice, 1 cup of mango and all the honey until the mixture becomes completely smooth. Divide into 4 glasses and refrigerate until ready to use. Rinse the blender.
2. Preheat the grill to medium-high heat. Mix the remaining cup of mango, ¼ cup water, ¼ cup vinegar, sultanas, olive oil, cayenne pepper, tomatoes and garlic in a microwave bowl. Cover with a piece of clear film and cook in the microwave until the tomatoes become soft, for about 3 minutes. Leave to cool slightly and pass in a blender. Transfer to a small bowl. Leave 2 tablespoons aside to garnish, turn the chicken into the remaining mixture.
3. Put the corn on the grill, cover and bake, turning it over if necessary, until it is burnt, about 10 minutes. Remove and keep warm.
4. Brush the grill over medium heat and brush the grills with a little oil. Turn the chicken legs into half the remaining sauce and ½ teaspoon of salt. Put on the grill and cook until the cooking marks appear and the internal temperature reaches 75°C on an instantaneous thermometer, 8 to 10 minutes per side. Bart and sprinkle a few times with the remaining sauce while cooking.
5. While the chicken is cooking, beat the remaining 2 tablespoons of yogurt, the 2 tablespoons of sauce set aside, the remaining spoonful of vinegar, 1 tablespoon of water and ¼ teaspoon of salt in a large bowl. Mix the mixed salad with the carrots. Divide chicken, corn and salad into 4 serving dishes. Garnish the salad with the dressing set aside. Serve each plate with a mango smoothie.

Nutrition:

Calories 346

Protein 56

Fat 45

Chinese Chicken Salad

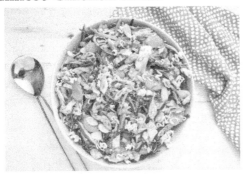

Preparation Time: 15 minutes

Cooking Time: 30 minutes

Servings: 4

Ingredients:

- For the chicken salad:
- 4 divided chicken breasts with skin and bones
- Olive oil of excellent quality
- Salt and freshly ground black pepper
- 500 g asparagus, with the ends removed and cut into three parts diagonally
- 1 red pepper, peeled
- Chinese condiment, recipe to follow
- 2 spring onions (both the white and the green part), sliced diagonally
- 1 tablespoon of white sesame seeds, toasted
- For Chinese dressing:
- 120 ml vegetable oil
- 60 ml of apple cider vinegar of excellent quality
- 60 ml soy sauce
- 1 ½ tablespoon of black sesame
- ½ tablespoon of honey
- 1 clove of garlic, minced
- ½ teaspoon of fresh peeled and grated ginger
- ½ tablespoon sesame seeds, toasted
- 60 g peanut butter
- 2 teaspoons of salt
- ½ teaspoons freshly ground black pepper

Directions:

1. For the chicken salad:
2. Heat the oven to 180°C (or 200°C for gas oven). Put the chicken breast on a baking tray and rub the skin with a little olive oil. Season freely with salt and pepper.
3. Brown for 35 to 40 minutes, until the chicken is freshly cooked. Let it cool down as long as it takes to handle it. Remove the meat from the bones, remove the skin and chop the chicken into medium-sized pieces.
4. Blanch the asparagus in a pot of salted water for 3-5 minutes until tender. Soak them in water with ice to stop cooking. Drain them. Cut the peppers into strips the same size as the asparagus. In a large bowl, mix the chopped chicken, asparagus and peppers.
5. Spread the Chinese dressing on chicken and vegetables. Add the spring onions and sesame seeds, and season to taste. Serve cold or at room temperature.
6. For Chinese dressing:
7. Mix all ingredients and set aside until use.

Nutrition:

Calories 222

Protein 28

Fat 10

Sugar 6

Chicken Salad

Preparation Time: 15 minutes
Cooking Time: 25 minutes
Servings: 4
Ingredients:

- For the Buffalo chicken salad:
- 2 chicken breasts (225 g) peeled, boned, cut in half
- 2 tablespoons of hot cayenne pepper sauce (or another type of hot sauce), plus an addition depending on taste
- 2 tablespoons of olive oil
- 2 romaine lettuce heart, cut into 2 cm strips
- 4 celery stalks, finely sliced
- 2 carrots, roughly grated
- 2 fresh onions, only the green part, sliced
- 125 ml of blue cheese dressing, recipe to follow
- For the seasoning of blue cheese
- 2 tablespoons mayonnaise
- 70 ml of partially skimmed buttermilk
- 70 ml low-fat white yoghurt
- 1 tablespoon of wine vinegar
- ½ teaspoon of sugar
- 35 g of chopped blue cheese
- Salt and freshly ground black pepper

Directions:

1. For the Buffalo chicken salad:
2. Preheat the grid.
3. Place the chicken between 2 sheets of baking paper and beat it with a meat tenderizer so that it is about 2 cm thick, then cut the chicken sideways creating 1 cm strips.
4. In a large bowl, add the hot sauce and oil, add the chicken and turn it over until it is well soaked. Place the chicken on a baking tray and grill until well cooked, about 4-6 minutes, turning it once.
5. In a large bowl, add the lettuce, celery, grated carrots and fresh onions. Add the seasoning of blue cheese. Distribute the vegetables in 4 plates and arrange the chicken on each of the dishes. Serve with hot sauce on the side.
6. For the blue cheese dressing:
7. Cover a small bowl with absorbent paper folded in four. Spread the yoghurt on the paper and put it in the fridge for 20 minutes to drain and firm it.
8. In a medium bowl, beat the buttermilk and firm yogurt with mayonnaise until well blended. Add the vinegar and sugar and keep beating until well blended. Add the blue cheese and season with salt and pepper to taste.

Nutrition:
321 calories
Fat 3
Fiber 5
Carbs 7
Protein 4

Tofu Meat and Salad

Preparation Time: 15 minutes
Cooking Time: 20 minutes
Servings: 3
Ingredients:

- 1 tablespoon of garlic sauce and chili in a bottle
- 1 1/2 tablespoon sesame oil
- 3 tablespoons of low-sodium soy sauce

- 60 ml hoisin sauce
- 2 tablespoons rice vinegar
- 2 tablespoons of sherry or Chinese cooking wine
- 225 g of extra-solid tofu
- 2 teaspoons of rapeseed oil
- 2 tablespoons of finely chopped fresh ginger
- 4 spring onions, with the green part chopped and set aside, in thin slices
- 225 g of minced lean beef (90% or more lean)
- 25 g of diced Chinese water chestnuts
- 1 large head of cappuccino lettuce, with the leaves separated, but without the outer ones
- 1 red pepper, diced

Directions:

- In a bowl, mix together the garlic and chili sauce, sesame oil, soy sauce, hoisin sauce, vinegar and sherry.
- Cut the tofu into 1 cm thick slices and place them on a kitchen towel. Use the cloth to dab the tofu well to remove as much water as possible. Should take a couple of minutes and about three dish towels. Chop the dry tofu well and set aside.
- Heat the oil in a wok or in a very large pan and medium flame. Add the ginger and the white part of the spring onions and cook until the spring onions become translucent and the ginger fragrant, for about 2-3 minutes. Add the beef and tofu and cook, stirring, until the meat becomes dull and freshly cooked, for about 4-5 minutes. Add the sauce set aside. Reduce the flame and simmer slowly, stirring, for another 3-4 minutes. Add

the chestnuts and mix well to incorporate.
- Fill each lettuce leaf with stuffing. Serve by decorating with the green part of the spring onions, red pepper and peanuts.

Nutrition:

Calories 122

Fat 2

Protein 66

Asparagus and Pistachios Vinaigrette

Preparation Time: 10 minutes

Cooking Time: 5minutes

Servings: 2

Ingredients:

- Two 455g bunches of large asparagus, without the tip
- 1 tablespoon of olive oil
- Salt and freshly ground black pepper
- 6 tablespoons of sliced pistachios blanched and boiled
- 1 1/2 tablespoon lemon juice
- 1/4 teaspoon of sugar
- 1 1/2 teaspoon lemon zest

Directions:

1. Preheat the oven to 220°C. Put the grill in the top third of the oven. Place the asparagus on a baking tray covered with baking paper. Sprinkle with olive oil and season with a little salt and pepper. Bake for 15 minutes, until soft.
2. Meanwhile, blend 5 tablespoons of almonds, lemon juice, sugar and 6 tablespoons of water for 1 minute until smooth. Taste and regulate salt.

Pour the sauce on a plate and put the spinach on the sauce. Decorate with peel and the remaining spoon of pistachios

Nutrition:

Calories 560

Fat 5

Fiber 2

Carbs 3

Protein 9

Turkey Meatballs

Preparation Time: 30 minutes

Cooking Time: 0 minutes

Servings: 4

Ingredients:

- 255g turkey sausage
- 2 tablespoons of extra virgin olive oil
- One can of 425g chickpeas, rinsed and drained...
- 1/2 medium onion, chopped, 2/3 cup
- 2 cloves of garlic, finely chopped
- 1 teaspoon of cumin
- 1/2 cup flour
- 1/2 teaspoon instant yeast for desserts
- Salt and ground black pepper
- 1 cup of Greek yogurt
- 2 tablespoons of lime juice
- 2 radicchio hearts, chopped
- Hot sauce

Directions:

1. Preheat the oven to 200°C.
2. In a processor, blend the chickpeas, onion, garlic, cumin, 1 teaspoon salt and 1/2 teaspoon pepper until all the ingredients are finely chopped. Add the flour, baking powder and blend to make everything mix well. Transfer to a medium bowl and add the sausage, stirring together with your hands. Cover and refrigerate for 30 minutes.
3. Once cold, take the mixture in spoonful, forming 1-inch balls with wet hands. Heat the olive oil in a pan over medium heat. In two groups, put the falafel in the pan and cook until slightly brown, about a minute and a half per side. Transfer to a baking tray and bake in the oven until well cooked, for about 10 minutes.
4. Mix together the yogurt, lime juice, 1/2 teaspoon salt and 1/4 teaspoon pepper. Divide the lettuce into 4 plates, season with some yogurt sauce.

Nutrition:

Calories 189

Fat 5

Protein 77

Sugar 3

Chicken, Bacon and Avocado Cloud Sandwiches

Preparation Time: 10 minutes

Cooking Time: 25 minutes

Servings: 6

Ingredients:

- For cloud bread
- 3 large eggs
- 4 oz. cream cheese
- ½ tablespoon. ground psyllium husk powder
- ½ teaspoon baking powder
- A pinch of salt
- To assemble sandwich

- 6 slices of bacon, cooked and chopped
- 6 slices pepper Jack cheese
- ½ avocado, sliced
- 1 cup cooked chicken breasts, shredded
- 3 tablespoons. mayonnaise

Directions:
1. Preheat your oven to 300 degrees.
2. Prepare a baking sheet by lining it with parchment paper.
3. Separate the egg whites and egg yolks, and place into separate bowls.
4. Whisk the egg whites until very stiff. Set aside.
5. Combined egg yolks and cream cheese.
6. Add the psyllium husk powder and baking powder to the egg yolk mixture. Gently fold in.
7. Add the egg whites into the egg mixture and gently fold in.
8. Dollop the mixture onto the prepared baking sheet to create 12 cloud bread. Use a spatula to spread the circles around to form ½-inch thick pieces gently.
9. Bake for 25 minutes or until the tops are golden brown.
10. Allow the cloud bread to cool completely before serving. Can be refrigerated for up to 3 days of frozen for up to 3 months. If food prepping, place a layer of parchment paper between each bread slice to avoid having them getting stuck together. Simply toast in the oven for 5 minutes when it is time to serve.
11. To assemble sandwiches, place mayonnaise on one side of one cloud bread. Layer with the remaining sandwich ingredients and top with another slice of cloud bread.

Nutrition:
Calories: 333 kcal Carbs: 5g
Fat: 26g Protein: 19.9g

Roasted Lemon Chicken Sandwich

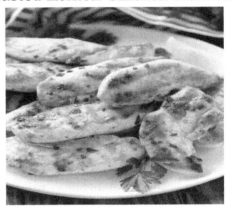

Preparation Time: 15 minutes
Cooking Time: 1 hour 30 minutes
Servings: 12
Ingredients:
- 1 kg whole chicken
- 5 tablespoons. butter
- 1 lemon, cut into wedges
- 1 tablespoon. garlic powder
- Salt and pepper to taste
- 2 tablespoons. mayonnaise
- Keto-friendly bread

Directions:
1. Preheat the oven to 350 degrees F.
2. Grease a deep baking dish with butter.
3. Ensure that the chicken is patted dry and that the gizzards have been removed.
4. Combine the butter, garlic powder, salt and pepper.
5. Rub the entire chicken with it, including in the cavity.

6. Place the lemon and onion inside the chicken and place the chicken in the prepared baking dish.

7. Bake for about 1½ hours, depending on the size of the chicken.

8. Baste the chicken often with the drippings. If the drippings begin to dry, add water. The chicken is done when a thermometer, insert it into the thickest part of the thigh reads 165 degrees F or when the clear juices run when the thickest part of the thigh is pierced.

9. Allow the chicken to cool before slicing.

10. To assemble sandwich, shred some of the breast meat and mix with the mayonnaise. Place the mixture between the two bread slices.

11. To save the chicken, refrigerated for up to 5 days or freeze for up to 1 month.

Nutrition:

Calories: 214 kcal Carbs: 1.6 g

Fat: 11.8 g Protein: 24.4 g.

Keto-Friendly Skillet Pepperoni Pizza

Preparation Time: 10 minutes

Cooking Time: 6 minutes

Servings: 4

Ingredients:

For Crust

½ cup almond flour

½ teaspoon baking powder

8 large egg whites, whisked into stiff peaks

Salt and pepper to taste

Toppings

3 tablespoons. Unsweetened tomato sauce

½ cup shredded cheddar cheese

½ cup pepperoni

Directions

Gently incorporate the almond flour into the egg whites. Ensure that no lumps remain.

Stir in the remaining crust ingredients.

Heat a nonstick skillet over medium heat. Spray with nonstick spray.

Pour the batter into the heated skillet to cover the bottom of the skillet.

Cover the skillet with a lid and cook the pizza crust to cook for about 4 minutes or until bubbles that appear on the top.

Flip the dough and add the toppings, starting with the tomato sauce and ending with the pepperoni

Cook the pizza for 2 more minutes.

Allow the pizza to cool slightly before serving.

Can be stored in the refrigerator for up to 5 days and frozen for up to 1 month.

Nutrition:

Calories: 175 kcal Carbs: 1.9 g

Fat: 12 g Protein: 14.3 g.

Cheesy Chicken Cauliflower

Preparation Time: 5 minutes

Cooking Time: 10 minutes

Servings: 4

Ingredients:

- 2 cups cauliflower florets, chopped
- ½ cup red bell pepper, chopped
- 1 cup roasted chicken, shredded (Lunch Recipes: Roasted Lemon Chicken Sandwich)
- ¼ cup shredded cheddar cheese
- 1 tablespoon. butter
- 1 tablespoon. sour cream

- Salt and pepper to taste

Directions:

1. Stir fry the cauliflower and peppers in the butter over medium heat until the veggies are tender.
2. Add the chicken and cook until the chicken is warmed through.
3. Add the remaining ingredients and stir until the cheese is melted.
4. Serve warm.

Nutrition:

Calories: 144 kcal Carbs: 4 g

Fat: 8.5 g Protein: 13.2 g.

Chicken Avocado Salad

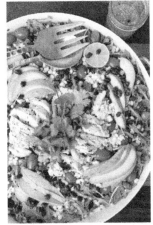

Preparation Time: 7 minutes

Cooking Time: 10 minutes

Servings: 4

Ingredients:

- 1 cup roasted chicken, shredded (Lunch Recipes: Roasted Lemon Chicken Sandwich)
- 1 bacon strip, cooked and chopped
- 1/2 medium avocado, chopped
- ¼ cup cheddar cheese, grated
- 1 hard-boiled egg, chopped

- 1 cup romaine lettuce, chopped
- 1 tablespoon. olive oil
- 1 tablespoon. apple cider vinegar
- Salt and pepper to taste

Directions:

1. Create the dressing by mixing apple cider vinegar, oil, salt and pepper.
2. Combine all the other ingredients in a mixing bowl.
3. Drizzle with the dressing and toss.
4. Can be refrigerated for up to 3 days.

Nutrition:

Calories: 220 kcal

Carbs: 2.8 g

Fat: 16.7 g

Protein: 14.8 g.

Chicken Broccoli Dinner

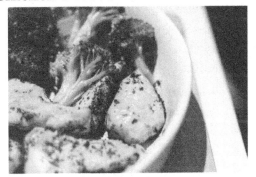

Preparation Time: 10 minutes

Cooking Time: 5 minutes

Servings: 1

Ingredients:

- 1 roasted chicken leg (Lunch Recipes: Roasted Lemon Chicken Sandwich)
- ½ cup broccoli florets
- ½ tablespoon. unsalted butter, softened
- 2 garlic cloves, minced
- Salt and pepper to taste

Directions:

1. Boil the broccoli in lightly salted water for 5 minutes. Drain the water from the pot and keep the broccoli in the pot. Keep the lid on to keep the broccoli warm.
2. Mix all the butter, garlic, salt and pepper in a small bowl to create garlic butter.
3. Place the chicken, broccoli and garlic butter.

Nutrition:

Calories: 257 kcal

Carbs: 5.1 g

Fat: 14 g

Protein: 27.4 g.

Easy Meatballs

Preparation Time: 10 minutes

Cooking Time: 20 minutes

Servings: 4

Ingredients:

- 1 lb. ground beef
- 1 egg, beaten
- Salt and pepper to taste
- 1 teaspoon garlic powder
- 1 teaspoon onion powder
- 2 tablespoons. butter
- ¼ cup mayonnaise
- ¼ cup pickled jalapeños
- 1 cup cheddar cheese, grated

Directions

1. Combine the cheese, mayonnaise, pickled jalapenos, salt, pepper, garlic powder and onion powder in a large mixing bowl.
2. Add the beef and egg and combine using clean hands.

3. Form large meatballs. Makes about 12.
4. Fry the meatballs in the butter over medium heat for about 4 minutes on each side or until golden brown.
5. Serve warm with a keto-friendly side.
6. The meatball mixture can also be used to make a meatloaf. Just preheat your oven to 400 degrees F, press the mixture into a loaf pan and bake for about 30 minutes or until the top is golden brown.
7. Can be refrigerated for up to 5 days or frozen for up to 3 months.

Nutrition:

Calories: 454 kcal

Carbs: 5 g

Fat: 28.2 g

Protein: 43.2 g.

Chicken Casserole

Preparation Time: 10 minutes

Cooking Time: 40 minutes

Servings: 8

Ingredients:

- 1 lb. boneless chicken breasts, cut into 1" cubes
- 2 tablespoons. butter
- 4 tablespoons. green pesto
- 1 cup heavy whipping cream
- ¼ cup green bell peppers, diced
- 1 cup feta cheese, diced
- 1 garlic clove, minced
- Salt and pepper to taste

Directions

1. Preheat your oven to 400 degrees F.

2. Season the chicken with salt and pepper then batch fry in the butter until golden brown.
3. Place the fried chicken pieces in a baking dish. Add the feta cheese, garlic and bell peppers.
4. Combine the pesto and heavy cream in a bowl. Pour on top of the chicken mixture and spread with a spatula.
5. Bake for 30 minutes or until the casserole is light brown around the edges.
6. Serve warm.
7. Can be refrigerated for up to 5 days and frozen for 2 weeks.

Nutrition:
Calories: 294 kcal
 Carbs: 1.7 g
Fat: 22.7 g
Protein: 20.1 g.

Lemon Baked Salmon

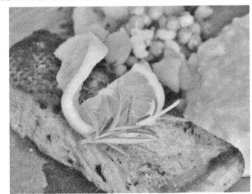

Preparation Time: 10 minutes
Cooking Time: 30 minutes
Servings: 4
Ingredients:

- 1 lb. salmon
- 1 tablespoon. olive oil
- Salt and pepper to taste

- 1 tablespoon. butter
- 1 lemon, thinly sliced
- 1 tablespoon. lemon juice

Directions:
1. Preheat your oven to 400 degrees F.
2. Grease a baking dish with the olive oil and place the salmon skin-side down.
3. Season the salmon with salt and pepper then top with the lemon slices.
4. Slice half the butter and place over the salmon.
5. Bake for 20minutes or until the salmon flakes easily.
6. Melt the remaining butter in a saucepan. When it starts to bubble, remove from heat and allow to cool before adding the lemon juice.
7. Drizzle the lemon butter over the salmon and Serve warm.

Nutrition:
Calories: 211 kcal
Carbs: 1.5 g
Fat: 13.5 g
Protein: 22.2 g.

Cauliflower Mash

Preparation Time: 10 minutes
Cooking Time: 5 minutes
Servings: 8
Ingredients:

- 4 cups cauliflower florets, chopped
- 1 cup grated parmesan cheese
- 6 tablespoons. butter
- ½ lemon, juice and zest
- Salt and pepper to taste

Directions:
1. Boil the cauliflower in lightly salted water over high heat for 5 minutes or

until the florets are tender but still firm.

2. Strain the cauliflower in a colander and add the cauliflower to a food processor
3. Add the remaining ingredients and pulse the mixture to a smooth and creamy consistency
4. Serve with protein like salmon, chicken or meatballs.
5. Can be refrigerated for up to 3 days.

Nutrition:

Calories: 101 kcal

Carbs: 3.1 g

Fat: 9.5 g

Protein: 2.2 g.

Roasted Chicken Soup

Preparation Time: 10 minutes

Cooking Time: 25 minutes

Servings: 6

Ingredients:

- 4 cups roasted chicken, shredded (Lunch Recipes: Roasted Lemon Chicken Sandwich)
- 2 tablespoons. butter
- 2 celery stalks, chopped
- 1 cup mushrooms, sliced
- 4 cups green cabbage, sliced into strips
- 2 garlic cloves, minced
- 6 cups chicken broth
- 1 carrot, sliced
- Salt and pepper to taste
- 1 tablespoon. garlic powder
- 1 tablespoon. onion powder

Directions:

1. Sauté the celery, mushrooms and garlic in the butter in a pot over medium heat for 4 minutes.
2. Add broth, carrots, garlic powder, onion powder, salt, and pepper.
3. Simmer for 10 minutes or until the vegetables are tender.
4. Add the chicken and cabbage and simmer for another 10 minutes or until the cabbage is tender.
5. Serve warm.
6. Can be refrigerated for up to 3 days or frozen for up to 1 month.

Nutrition:

Calories: 279 kcal

Carbs: 7.5 g

Fat: 12.3 g

Protein: 33.4 g.

CHAPTER 3:

Dinner Recipes

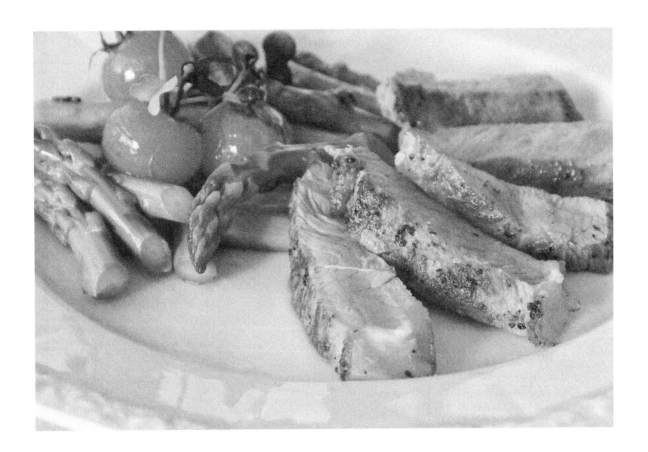

Cheesy Salmon & Asparagus

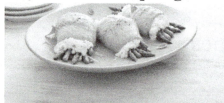

Preparation Time: 15 minutes

Cooking Time: 15 Minutes

Servings: 4

Ingredients:

- 4 Salmon Fillets, 6 Ounces Each & Skin On
- 2 lbs. Asparagus, Trimmed
- 6 Tablespoons Butter
- 4 Cloves Garlic, Minced
- ½ Cup Parmesan Cheese, Grated
- Sea Salt & Black Pepper to Taste

Directions:

1. Start by heating your oven to 400, lining a baking sheet with foil.
2. Pat your salmon dry, seasoning with salt and pepper.
3. Put your salmon in a pan, arranging your asparagus around it.
4. Put a saucepan over medium heat and melt your butter. Add in your garlic, stirring until it browns which takes about three minutes. Drizzle this butter over your salmon and asparagus.
5. Top with parmesan cheese and then cook for twelve minutes. Broil for another three before serving warm.

Nutrition:

Calories: 434 Protein: 42 Grams

Fat: 26 Grams Net Carbs: 6 Grams

Herb Pork Chops

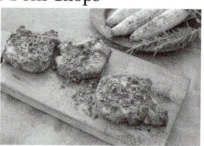

Preparation Time: minutes

Cooking Time: 30 Minutes

Servings: 4

Ingredients:

- 2 Tablespoons Butter + More for Coating
- 4 Pork Chops, Boneless
- 2 Tablespoons Italian Seasoning
- 2 Tablespoons Italian Leaf Parsley Chopped
- 2 Tablespoons Olive Oil
- Sea Salt & Black Pepper to Taste

Directions:

1. Start by heating your oven to 350 and coat a baking dish with butter.
2. Season your pork chops, and then top with fresh parsley, drizzling with olive oil and a half a tablespoon of butter each to bake.
3. Bake for twenty to twenty-five minutes.

Nutrition:

Calories: 333

Protein: 31 Grams

Fat: 23 Grams

Net Carbs: 0 Grams

Paprika Chicken

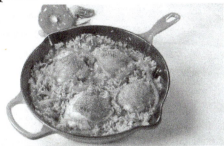

Preparation Time: 15 minutes

Cooking Time: 20 Minutes

Servings: 4

Ingredients:

- 2 Teaspoons Smoked Paprika
- ½ Cup Heavy Whipping Cream
- ½ Cup Sweet Onion, Chopped
- 1 Tablespoon Olive Oil
- 4 Chicken Breasts, Skin On & 4 Ounces Each
- ½ Cup Sour Cream
- 2 Tablespoons Parsley, Chopped

Directions:

1. Season your chicken with salt and pepper, putting a skillet over medium-high heat. Add your oil, and once it simmers, sear your chicken on both sides. It should take about fifteen minutes to cook your chicken all the way through. Put your chicken to the side.
2. Add in your onion, sautéing for four minutes or until tender.
3. Stir in your paprika and cream, bringing it to a simmer.
4. Return your chicken to the skillet, simmering for five more minutes.
5. Stir in sour cream and serve topped with parsley.

Nutrition:

Calories: 389

Protein: 25 Grams

Fat: 30 Grams

Net Carbs: 4 Grams

Coconut Chicken

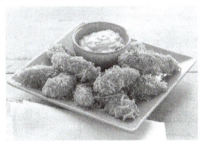

Preparation Time: 10 minutes

Cooking Time: 30 Minutes

Servings: 4

Ingredients:

- 1 Teaspoon Ground Cumin
- 1 Teaspoon Ground Coriander
- ¼ Cup Cilantro, Fresh & Chopped
- 1 Cup Coconut Milk
- 1 Tablespoon Curry Powder
- ½ Cup Sweet Onion, Chopped
- 2 Tablespoons Olive Oil
- 4 Chicken Breasts, 4 Ounces Each & Cut into 2 Inch Chunks

Directions:

1. Get out a saucepan, adding in your oil and heating it over medium-high heat.
2. Sauté your chicken until it's almost completely cooked, which will take roughly ten minutes.
3. Add in your onion, cooking for another three minutes.

4. Whisk your curry powder, coconut milk, coriander and cumin together.
5. Pour the sauce into your pan, bringing it to a boil with your chicken.
6. Reduce the heat, and let it simmer for ten minutes.
7. Serve topped with cilantro.

Nutrition:

Calories: 382

Protein: 23 Grams

Fat: 31 Grams

Net Carbs: 4 Grams

Cabbage & Chicken Plates

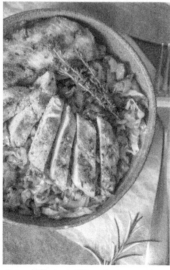

Preparation Time: 25 minutes

Cooking Time: 0 Minutes

Servings: 4

Ingredients:

- 1 Cup Bean Sprouts, Fresh
- 2 Tablespoons Sesame & Garlic Flavored Oil
- ½ Cup Onion, Sliced
- 4 Cups Bok Choy, Shredded
- 3 Stalks Celery, Chopped
- 1 Tablespoon Ginger, Minced
- 2 Tablespoon Coconut Aminos
- 1 Teaspoon Stevia
- 1 Cup Chicken Broth
- 1 ½ Teaspoons Minced Garlic
- 1 Teaspoon Arrowroot
- 4 Chicken Breasts, Boneless, Cooked & Sliced Thin

Directions:

1. Shred your cabbage, and then add your chicken and onion together.
2. Add in a dollop of mayonnaise if desired, drizzling with oil
3. Season as desired and serve.

Nutrition:

Calories: 368 Protein: 42 Grams

Fat: 18 Grams

Net Carbs: 8 Grams

Grilled Chicken & Cheesy Spinach

Preparation Time: 7minutes

Cooking Time: 6 Minutes

Servings: 6

Ingredients:

- 3 Ounces Mozzarella Cheese, Part Skim
- 3 Chicken Breasts, Large & Sliced in Half
- 10 Ounces Spinach, Frozen, Thawed & Drained
- ½ Cup Roasted Red Peppers, Sliced into Strips
- 2 Cloves Garlic Minced
- 1 Teaspoon Olive Oil
- Sea Salt & Black Pepper to Taste

Directions:

1. Start by heating your oven to 400, and then grease a pan.
2. Bake your chicken breasts for two to three minutes per side.
3. In another skillet, cook your garlic and spinach in oil for three minutes.
4. Put your chicken on a pan, topping it with spinach, roasted peppers and mozzarella.
5. Bake until your cheese melts and serve warm.

Nutrition:

Calories: 195

Protein: 30 Grams

Fat: 7 Grams

Net Carbs: 3 Grams

Balsamic Chicken with Vegetables

Preparation Time: 15 minutes

Cooking Time: 25 Minutes

Servings: 4

Ingredients:

- 8 chicken Cutlets, Skinless & Boneless
- ½ Cup Buttermilk, Low Fat
- 4 Tablespoons Dijon Mustard
- 2/3 Cup Almond Meal
- 2/3 Cup Cashews Chopped
- 4 Teaspoons Stevia
- ¾ Teaspoon Rosemary
- Sea Salt & Black Pepper to Taste

Directions:

1. Start by heating your oven to 425.
2. Mix your buttermilk and mustard together in a bowl
3. Add your chicken, coating it.

4. Put a skillet over medium heat, and then add in your almond meal. Bake until its golden, putting it in a bowl.
5. Add your sea salt, pepper, rosemary and cashews, mixing well. Coat your chicken with the almond meal mix, and then put it in a baking pan.
6. Bake for twenty-five minutes.

Nutrition:

Calories: 248

Protein: 27 Grams

Fat: 8 Grams Net

Carbs: 14 Grams

Steak & Broccoli Medley

Preparation Time: 10 minutes

Cooking Time: 10 Minutes

Servings: 4

Ingredients:

- 4 Ounces Butter
- ¾ lb. Ribeye Steak
- 9 Ounces Broccoli
- 1 Yellow Onion
- 1 Tablespoon Coconut Aminos
- 1 Tablespoon Pumpkin Seeds
- Sea Salt & Black Pepper as Needed

Directions:

1. Slice your onion and steak before chopping your broccoli.
2. Put a frying pan over medium heat, adding in butter. Let it melt, and then add meat. Season with salt and pepper, placing your meat to the side.
3. Brown your onion and broccoli, adding more butter as necessary.

4. Add in your coconut aminos before adding your meat back.
5. Serve topped with pumpkin seeds and butter.

Nutrition:

Calories: 875

Protein: 40 Grams

Fat: 75 Grams Net

Carbs: 10 Grams

Stuffed Meat Loaf

Preparation Time: 20 minutes

Cooking Time: 1 Hour

Servings: 8

Ingredients:

- 17 Ounces Ground Beef
- ¼ Cup Onions, Diced
- 6 Slices Cheddar Cheese
- ¼ Cup Green Onions, Diced
- ½ Cup Spinach
- ¼ Cup Mushrooms

Directions:

1. Mix your salt, pepper, meat, cumin and garlic together before greasing a pan.
2. Put your cheese on the bottom of your meatloaf, adding in the spinach, mushrooms and onions, and then use leftover meat to cover the top.
3. Bake at 350 for an hour before serving.

Nutrition:

Calories: 248

Protein: 15 Grams

Fat: 20 Grams

Net Carbs: 1 Gram

Beef Cabbage Rolls

Preparation Time: 20 minutes

Cooking Time: 6 Hours 10 Minutes

Servings: 5

Ingredients:

- 3 ½ lb. Corned Beef
- 15 Cabbage Leaves, Large
- 1 Onion
- 1 Lemon
- ¼ Cup Coffee
- ¼ Cup White Wine
- 1 Tablespoon Bacon Fat, Rendered
- 1 Tablespoon Brown Mustard
- 2 Tablespoons Himalayan Pink Sea Salt
- 2 Tablespoons Worcestershire Sauce
- 1 Teaspoon Whole Peppercorns
- 1 Teaspoon Mustard Seeds
- ½ Teaspoon Red Pepper Flakes
- ¼ Teaspoons Cloves
- ¼ Teaspoon Allspice
- 1 Bay Leaf, Large

Directions:

1. Add your liquids, corned beef and spices into a slow cooker, cooking on low for six hours.
2. Bring a pot of water to a boil, adding your cabbage leaves and one sliced onion, bringing it to a boil for three minutes.
3. Remove your cabbage, putting it in ice water for three to four minutes, continuing to boil your onion.

4. Dry the leaves off, slicing your meat, and adding in your cooked onion and meat into your leaves.

Nutrition:

Calories: 481 Protein: 35 Grams

Fat: 25 Grams Net Carbs: 4 Grams

Zucchini Fettuccine with Beef

Preparation Time: 15 minutes

Cooking Time: 30 minutes

Servings: 4

Ingredients:

- 15 oz. ground beef
- 3 tbsp butter
- 1 yellow onion
- 8 oz. mushrooms
- 1 tbsp dried thyme
- ½ tsp salt
- 1 pinch ground black pepper
- 8 oz. blue cheese
- 1½ cups sour cream

Zucchini fettuccine:

- 2 zucchinis
- 1 oz. olive oil or butter
- Salt and pepper

Directions:

1. Peel the onion and chop it finely.
2. Melt the butter and sauté the onion until the onions are softened and transparent.
3. Add the ground beef and fry this for a few more minutes with the onion until it is browned and cooked through.
4. Slice or dice the mushrooms, and add it to the ground beef. Sauté the mushrooms with the beef mixture for a few minutes more, or until lightly brown.

5. Season it with thyme, salt, and pepper. Crumble the cheese over the hot mixture. Stir it well.
6. Add the sour cream and bring the mixture to a light boil. Lower the heat to a medium-low setting and let it simmer for about 10 minutes.

Zucchini fettuccine:

1. Calculate about one medium-sized zucchini per person.
2. Slice the zucchini lengthwise in half.
3. Scoop out the seeds with a spoon and slice the halves super thinly, lengthwise (julienne) with a potato peeler, or you can use a spiralizer to make zoodles (zucchini noodles.)
4. Toss the zucchini in some hot sauce of your choice and serve it immediately.
5. If you are not going to be serving your zucchini with a hot sauce, then boil half a gallon of salted water in a large pot and parboil the zucchini slices for a minute. This makes them easier to eat
6. Drain the water from the pot and add some olive oil or a knob of butter. Salt and pepper to taste.

Nutrition:

Calories: 456 Protein: 32 Grams

Fat: 15 Grams Net Carbs: 13 Gram

Oven-Baked Chicken in Garlic Butter

Preparation Time: 25 minutes

Cooking Time: 1 hour 30 minutes

Servings: 3

Ingredients:

- 3 lbs. chickens, a whole bird

- 2 tsp sea salt
- ½ tsp ground black pepper
- 51/3 oz. butter
- 2 garlic cloves, minced

Directions:

1. Preheat the oven to 400°F.
2. Season the chicken with salt and pepper, both inside and out.
3. The chicken must go breast side up in the baking dish.
4. Combine the garlic and butter in a saucepan over a medium heat. The butter should not turn brown or burn, just melt it gently.
5. Let the butter cool down once it is melted.
6. Pour the garlic butter mixture all over and inside the chicken. Bake the chicken on the lower oven rack for 1 to1 ½ hours, or until internal temperature reaches 180°F. Baste it with the juices from the bottom of the pan every 20 minutes.
7. Serve with the juices.

Nutrition:

Calories: 148
Protein: 39 Grams
Fat: 24 Grams
Net Carbs: 16 Gram

Keto Chicken Garam Masala

Preparation Time: 10 minutes
Cooking Time: 20 minutes
Servings: 4
Ingredients:

- 25 oz. chicken breasts
- 3 tbsp butter or ghee
- Salt

- 1 red bell pepper, finely diced
- 1¼ cups coconut cream or heavy whipping cream
- 1 tbsp fresh parsley, finely chopped
- Garam masala:
- 1 tsp ground cumin
- 1 - 2 tsp coriander seed, ground
- 1 tsp ground cardamom (green)
- 1 tsp turmeric, ground
- 1 tsp ground ginger
- 1 tsp paprika powder
- 1 tsp chili powder
- 1 pinch ground nutmeg

Directions:

1. Preheat the oven to 400°F.
2. Mix the spices together for the Garam masala.
3. Cut the chicken breasts lengthwise. Place a large skillet over medium-high heat and fry the chicken in the butter until it is golden-brown.
4. Add half of the garam masala spice mix to the pan and stir it thoroughly.
5. Season with some salt, and place the chicken and all of the juices, into a baking dish.
6. Finely chop the bell pepper and add it to a bowl along with the coconut cream and the remaining half of the garam masala spice mix.
7. Pour over the chicken. Bake for 20 minutes.
8. Garnish with parsley and serve.

Nutrition:

Calories: 312 Protein: 21 Grams
Fat: 14 Grams Net Carbs: 2 Gram

Keto Lasagna

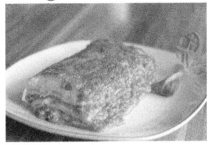

Preparation Time: 25 minutes

Cooking Time: 1 hour minutes

Servings: 4

Ingredients:

- 2 tbsp olive oil
- 1 yellow onion
- 1 garlic clove
- 20 oz. ground beef
- 3 tbsp tomato paste
- ½ tbsp dried basil
- 1 tsp salt
- ¼ tsp ground black pepper
- ½ cup water
- Keto pasta
- 8 eggs
- 10 oz. cream cheese
- 1 tsp salt
- 5 tbsp ground psyllium husk powder

Cheese topping:

- 2 cups crème fraiche or sour cream
- 5 oz. shredded cheese
- 2 oz. grated parmesan cheese
- ½ tsp salt
- ¼ tsp ground black pepper
- ½ cup fresh parsley, finely chopped

Directions:

1. Start with the ground beef mixture.

2. Peel and finely chop the onion and the garlic. Fry them in olive oil until they are soft. Add the ground beef to the onion and garlic and cook until it is golden. Add the tomato paste and remaining spices.

3. Stir the mixture thoroughly and add some water. Bring it to a boil, turn the heat down, and let it simmer for at least 15 minutes, or until the majority of the water has evaporated. The lasagna sheets used don't soak up as much liquid as regular ones, so the mixture should be quite dry.

4. While that is happening, make the lasagna sheets according to the instructions that follow below.

5. Preheat the oven to 400°F. Mix the shredded cheese with sour cream and the Parmesan cheese. Reserve one or two tablespoons of the cheese aside for the topping. Add salt and pepper for taste and stir in the parsley.

6. Place the lasagna sheets and pasta sauce in layers in a greased baking dish.

7. Spread the crème fraiche mixture and the reserved Parmesan cheese on top.

8. Bake the lasagna in the oven for around 30 minutes or until the lasagna has a nicely browned surface. Serve with a green salad and a light dressing.

Lasagna sheets:

1. Preheat the oven to 300°F.

2. Add the eggs, cream cheese, and the salt to a mixing bowl and

blend into a smooth batter. Continue to whisk this while adding in the ground psyllium husk powder, just a little bit at a time. Let it sit for a few minutes.

3. Using a spatula spread the batter onto a baking sheet that is lined with parchment paper. Place more parchment paper on top and flatten it with a rolling pin until the mixture is at least 13" x 18". You can also divide it into two separate batches and use a different baking sheet for even thinner pasta.

4. Let the pieces of parchment paper stay in place. Bake the pasta for about 10 to12 minutes. Let it cool and remove the paper. Slice into sheets.

Nutrition:

Calories: 128

Protein: 25 Grams

Fat: 15 Grams

Net Carbs: 4 Gram

Keto Buffalo Drumsticks and Chili Aioli

Preparation Time: 12 minutes

Cooking Time: 40 minutes

Servings: 6

Ingredients:

- 2 lbs. chicken drumsticks or chicken wings
- 2 tbsp olive oil or coconut oil
- 2 tbsp white wine vinegar
- 1 tbsp tomato paste
- 1 tsp salt
- 1 tsp paprika powder

- 1 tablespoon Tabasco
- Butter or olive oil, for greasing the baking dish

Chili aioli:

- 2/3 cup mayonnaise
- 1 tablespoon smoked paprika powder or smoked chili powder
- 1 garlic clove, minced

Directions:

1. Preheat the oven to 450° (220°C).
2. Put the drumsticks in a plastic bag.
3. Mix the ingredients for the marinade and pour into the plastic bag. Shake the bag and let marinate for 10 minutes.
4. Coat a baking dish with oil. Place the drumsticks in the baking bowl and let bake for 30–40 minutes or until they are done and have turned a beautiful color.
5. Mix together mayonnaise, garlic, and chili.

Nutrition:

Calories: 409

Protein: 22 Grams

Fat: 10 Grams

Net Carbs: 6 Gram

Keto Fish Casserole

Preparation Time: 10 minutes

Cooking Time: 20 minutes

Servings: 4

Ingredients:

- 2 tbsp olive oil
- 15 oz. broccoli
- 6 scallions
- 2 tbsp small capers

- 1/6 oz. butter, for greasing the casserole dish
- 25 oz. white fish, in serving-sized pieces
- 1¼ cups heavy whipping cream
- 1 tbsp Dijon mustard
- 1 tsp salt
- ¼ tsp ground black pepper
- 1 tbsp dried parsley
- 3 oz. butter

Directions:

1. Preheat the oven to 400°F.
2. Divide the broccoli into smaller floret heads and include the stems. Peel it with a sharp knife or a potato peeler if the stem is rough or leafy.
3. Fry the broccoli florets in oil on a medium-high heat for about 5 minutes, until they are golden and soft. Season with salt and pepper to taste.
4. Add finely chopped scallions and the capers. Fry this for another 1 to 2 minutes and place the vegetables in a baking dish that has been greased.
5. Place the fish tightly in amongst the vegetables.
6. Mix the parsley, whipping cream and mustard together. Pour this over the fish and vegetables. Top it with slices of butter.
7. Bake the fish until it is cooked through, and it flakes easily with a fork. Serve as is, or with a tasty green salad.

Nutrition:

Calories: 314

Protein: 20 Grams

Fat: 8 Grams

Net Carbs: 5 Gram

Slow Cooker Keto Pork Roast

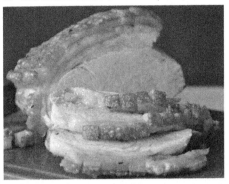

Preparation Time: 35 minutes

Cooking Time: 8 hours 20 minutes

Servings: 4

Ingredients:

- 30 oz. pork shoulder or pork roast
- ½ tbsp salt
- 1 bay leaf
- 5 black pep
- percorns
- 2½ cups water
- 2 tsp dried thyme or dried rosemary
- 2 garlic cloves
- 1½ oz. fresh ginger
- 1 tbsp olive oil or coconut oil
- 1 tbsp paprika powder
- ½ tsp ground black pepper

Creamy gravy:

- 1½ cups heavy whipping cream
- Juices from the roast

Directions:

1. Preheat the oven to a low heat of 200°F.
2. Season the meat with salt and place it into a deep baking dish.
3. Add water. Add a bay leaf, peppercorns, and thyme for more seasoning. Place the baking bowl in

the oven for 7 to 8 hours and cover it with aluminum foil.

4. If you are using a slow cooker for this, do the same process as in step 2, only add 1 cup of water. Cook it for 8 hours on low or for 4 hours on high setting.

5. Take the meat out of the baking dish, and reserve the pan juices in a separate pan to make gravy.

6. Turn the oven up to 450°F.

7. Finely chop or press the garlic and ginger into a small bowl. Add the oil, herbs, and pepper and stir well to combine together.

8. Rub the meat with the garlic and herb mixture.

9. Return the meat back to the baking dish, and roast it for about 10 to 15 minutes or until it looks golden-brown.

10. Cut the meat into thin slices to serve it with the creamy gravy and a fibrous vegetable side dish

Gravy:

1. Strain the reserved pan juices to get rid of any solid pieces from the liquid. Boil and reduce the pan juices to about half the original volume, this should be about 1 cup.

2. Pour the reduction into a pot with the whipping cream. Bring this to a boil. Reduce the heat and let it simmer to your desired consistency for a creamy gravy.

Nutrition:

Calories: 432

Protein: 15 Grams

Fat: 29 Grams

Net Carbs: 13 Gram

Fried Eggs with Kale and Pork

Preparation Time: 15 minutes

Cooking Time: 20 minutes

Servings: 5

Ingredients:

- ½ lb. kale
- 3 oz. butter
- 6 oz. smoked pork belly or bacon
- ¼ cup frozen cranberries
- 1 oz. pecans or walnuts
- 4 eggs
- Salt and pepper

Directions:

1. Cut and chop the kale into large squares. You can use pre-washed baby kale as a shortcut if you want. Melt two-thirds of the butter in a frying pan, and fry the kale on high heat until it is slightly browned around its edges.

2. Remove the kale from the frying pan and put it aside. Sear the pork belly in the same frying pan until it is crispy.

3. Turn the heat down. Put the sautéed kale back into the pan and add the cranberries and nuts. Stir this mixture until it is warmed through. Put it into a bowl on the side.

4. Turn up the heat once more, and fry the eggs in the remaining amount of the butter. Add salt and pepper to taste. Serve the eggs and greens immediately.

Nutrition:

Calories: 180

Protein: 23 Grams

Fat: 30 Grams

Net Carbs: 13 Gram

Cauliflower Soup with Pancetta

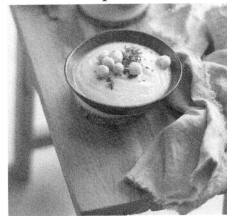

Preparation Time: 15 minutes

Cooking Time: 35 minutes

Servings: 4

Ingredients:

- 4 cups chicken broth or vegetable stock
- 15 oz. cauliflower
- 7 oz. cream cheese
- 1 tbsp Dijon mustard
- 4 oz. butter
- Salt and pepper
- 7 oz. pancetta or bacon, diced
- 1 tbsp butter, for frying
- 1 teaspoon paprika powder or smoked chili powder
- 3 oz. pecans

Directions:

1. Trim the cauliflower and cut it into smaller floret heads. The smaller the florets are, the quicker the soup will be ready.
2. Put aside a handful of the fresh cauliflower and chop into small 1/4 inch bits.
3. Sauté the finely chopped cauliflower and pancetta in butter until it is crispy. Add some nuts and the paprika powder at the end. Set aside the mixture for serving.
4. Boil the cauliflower until they are soft. Add the cream cheese, mustard, and butter.
5. Stir the soup well, using an immersion blender, to get to the desired consistency. The creamier the soup will become the longer you blend. Salt and pepper the soup to taste.
6. Serve soup in bowls, and top it with the fried pancetta mixture.

Nutrition:

Calories: 112

Protein: 10 Grams

Fat: 22 Grams

Net Carbs: 21 Gram

Butter Mayonnaise

Preparation Time: 20 minutes

Cooking Time: 25 minutes

Servings: 4

Ingredients:

- 51/3 oz. butter
- 1 egg yolk
- 1 tbsp Dijon mustard
- 1 tsp lemon juice
- ¼ tsp salt
- 1 pinch ground black pepper

Directions:

1. Melt the butter in a small saucepan. Pour it into a small pitcher or a jug with a spout and let the butter cool.
2. Mix together egg yolks and mustard in a small-sized bowl. Pour the butter in a thin stream while beating it with a hand mixer. Leave the sediment that settles at the bottom.

3. Keep beating the mixture until the mayonnaise turns thick and creamy. Add some lemon juice. Season it with salt and black pepper. Serve this immediately.

Nutrition:

Calories: 428

Protein: 45 Grams

Fat: 4 Grams

Net Carbs: 14 Gram

Meatloaf Wrapped in Bacon

Preparation Time: 10 minutes

Cooking Time: 15 minutes

Servings: 3

Ingredients:

- 2 tbsp butter
- 1 yellow onion, finely chopped
- 25 oz. ground beef or ground lamb/pork
- ½ cup heavy whipping cream
- ½ cup shredded cheese
- 1 egg
- 1 tbsp dried oregano or dried basil
- 1 tsp salt
- ½ tsp ground black pepper
- 7 oz. sliced bacon
- 1¼ cups heavy whipping cream, for the gravy

Directions:

1. Preheat the oven to 400°F.
2. Fry the onion until it is soft but not overly browned.
3. Mix the ground meat in a bowl with all the other ingredients, minus the bacon. Mix it well, but avoid overworking it as you do not want the mixture to become dense.
4. Mold the meat into a loaf shape and place it in a baking dish. Wrap the loaf completely in the bacon.
5. Bake the loaf in the middle rack of the oven for about 45 minutes. If you notice that the bacon begins to overcook before the meat is done, cover it with some aluminum foil and lower the heat a bit since you do not want burnt bacon.
6. Save all the juices that have accumulated in the baking dish from the meat and bacon, and use to make the gravy. Mix these juices and the cream in a smaller saucepan for the gravy.
7. Bring it to a boil and lower the heat and let it simmer for 10 to 15 minutes until it has the right consistency and is not lumpy.
8. Serve the meatloaf.
9. Serve with freshly boiled broccoli or some cauliflower with butter, salt, and pepper.

Nutrition:

Calories: 308

Protein: 21 Grams

Fat: 8 Grams

Net Carbs: 19 Gram

Keto Salmon with Broccoli Mash

Preparation Time: 20 minutes

Cooking Time: 15 minutes

Servings: 5

Ingredients:

Salmon burgers:

- 1½ lbs. salmon
- 1 egg
- ½ yellow onion

- 1 tsp salt
- ½ tsp pepper
- 2 oz. butter, for frying
- Green mash
- 1 lb. broccoli
- 5 oz. butter
- 2 oz. grated parmesan
- Salt and pepper

Lemon butter:

- 4 oz. butter at room temperature
- 2 tablespoons lemon juice
- Salt and pepper to taste

Directions:

1. Preheat the oven to 220° F. Cut the fish into smaller pieces and place them along with the rest of the ingredients for the burger, into a food processor.
2. Blend it for 30 to 45 seconds until you have a rough mixture. Don't mix it too thoroughly as you do not want tough burgers.
3. Shape 6 to 8 burgers and fry them for 4 to 5 minutes on each side on a medium heat in a generous amount of butter. Or even oil if you prefer. Keep them warm in the oven.
4. Trim the broccoli and cut it into smaller florets. You can use the stems as well just peel them and chop it into small pieces.
5. Bring a pot of salted water to a boil and add the broccoli to this. Cook it for a few minutes until it is soft, but not until all the texture is gone. Drain and discard the water used for boiling.
6. Use an immersion blender or even a food processor to mix the broccoli with the butter and the parmesan cheese. Season the broccoli mash to taste with salt and pepper.

7. Make the lemon butter by mixing room temperature butter with lemon juice, salt and pepper into a small bowl using electric beaters.
8. Serve the warm burgers with the side of green broccoli mash and a melting dollop of fresh lemon butter on top of the burger.

Nutrition:

Calories: 156

Protein: 15 Grams

Fat: 11 Grams

Net Carbs: 5 Gram

Oven Baked Sausage and Vegetables

Preparation Time: 10 minutes

Cooking Time: 25 minutes

Servings: 2

Ingredients:

- 1 oz. butter, for greasing the baking dish
- 1 small zucchini
- 2 yellow onions
- 3 garlic cloves
- 51/3 oz. tomatoes
- 7 oz. fresh mozzarella
- Sea salt
- Black pepper
- 1 tbsp dried basil
- Olive oil
- 1 lb. sausages in links, in links

For **Servings:**

- 1/2 cup mayonnaise

Directions:

1. Preheat the oven to 400°F. Grease the baking dish with butter.

2. Divide the zucchini into bite-sized pieces. Peel and cut the onion into wedges. Slice or chop the garlic.

3. Place zucchini, onions, garlic, and tomatoes in the baking dish. Dice the cheese and place among the vegetables. Season with salt, pepper and basil.

4. Sprinkle olive oil over the vegetables, and top with sausage.

5. Bake until the sausages are thoroughly cooked and the vegetables are browned.

6. Serve with a dollop of mayonnaise.

Nutrition:

Calories: 176

Protein: 31 Grams

Fat: 12 Grams

Net Carbs: 10 Gram

Keto Avocado Quiche

Preparation Time: 15 minutes

Cooking Time: 10 minutes

Servings: 4

Ingredients:

- Pie crust
- ¾ cup almond flour
- 4 tbsp sesame seeds
- 4 tbsp coconut flour
- 1 tbsp ground psyllium husk powder
- 1 tsp baking powder
- 1 pinch salt
- 3 tbsp olive oil or coconut oil
- 1 egg
- 4 tbsp water

Filling:

- 2 avocados, ripe
- Mayonnaise

- 3 eggs
- 2tbspfinely chopped fresh cilantro
- 1 finely chopped red chili
- Onion powder
- Salt
- ½ cup cream cheese
- 1¼ cups shredded cheese

Directions:

1. Preheat the oven to 350° F. Mix all the ingredients together for the pie dough in a food processor until the dough forms into a ball, this takes a few minutes usually. Use your hands or a fork in the absence of a food processor to knead the dough together.

2. Place a piece of parchment paper to a springform pan, no larger than 12 inches around. The springform pan makes it easier to take the pie out when it is done. Grease the pan and the parchment paper.

3. Using an oiled spatula or oil coated fingers, spread the dough into the pan. Bake the crust for 10 minutes.

4. Split the avocado in half. Remove the peel and pit it, and dice the avocado.

5. Take the seeds out from the chili and chop the chili very finely. Combine the avocado and the chili in a bowl and mix them together with the other ingredients.

6. Pour the mixture into the pie crust and bake it for 35 minutes or until it is a light golden brown. Serve it with a green salad.

Nutrition:

Calories: 323 Protein: 45 Grams

Fat: 18 Grams

Net Carbs: 10 Gram

Keto Berry Mousse

Preparation Time: 10 minutes

Cooking Time: 20 minutes

Servings: 4

Ingredients:

- 2 cups heavy whipping cream
- 3 oz. fresh raspberries, strawberries or even blueberries
- 2 oz. chopped pecans
- ½ lemon the zest
- ¼ tsp vanilla extract

Directions:

1. Pour the cream into a bowl and whip it with a hand mixer until soft peaks form. You can use an old whip too, but this will take some time. Add the lemon zest and vanilla once you are almost done whipping the cream mixture.
2. Combine berries and nuts into the whipped cream and stir it thoroughly.
3. Cover the mousse with plastic wrap and let it sit in the refrigerator for 3 or more hours for a firmer mousse. If your goal is to have a less firm consistency, you can eat the dessert right away.

Nutrition:

Calories: 105 Protein: 33 Grams

Fat: 14 Grams

Net Carbs: 20 Gram

Cinnamon Crunch Balls

Preparation Time: 5 minutes

Cooking Time: 10 minutes

Servings: 1

Ingredients:

- Unsalted butter

- Unsweetened shredded coconut
- Groundgreen cardamom
- Vanilla extract
- Ground cinnamon

Directions:

1. Bring the butter to room temperature.
2. Roast the shredded coconut carefully until they turn a little brown.
3. Mix the butter, half of the coconut and spices.
4. Form into walnut-sized balls. Roll in the rest of the coconut.
5. Store in refrigerator or freezer.

Nutrition:

Calories: 432

Protein: 23 Grams

Fat: 3 Grams

Net Carbs: 5 Gram

Keto Cheesecake and Blueberries

Preparation Time: 15 minutes

Cooking Time: 60 minutes

Servings: 2

Ingredients:

Crust:

- 1¼ cups almond flour
- 2 oz. butter
- 2 tbsperythritol
- ½ tsp vanilla extract

Filling:

- 20 oz. cream cheese
- ½ cup heavy whipping cream or crème fraiche
- 2 eggs
- 1 egg yolk
- 1 tsp lemon, zest
- ½ tsp vanilla extract

- 2 oz. fresh blueberries (optional)

Directions:

1. Preheat the oven to 350°F.
2. Butter a 9-inch springform and line the base of it with parchment paper.
3. Next, melt the butter for the crust and heat it until it lets off a nutty scent. This will give the crust an almost toffee-like flavor.
4. Remove it from the heat and add the almond flour, and vanilla. Combine these into firm dough and press the dough into the base of the pan. Bake for about 8 minutes, until the crust turns lightly golden. Set the crust aside and allow it to cool while you prepare the filling.
5. Combine together cream cheese, heavy cream, eggs, lemon zest, and the vanilla. Combine these ingredients well and make sure there are no lumps. Pour this cheese mixture over the crust.
6. Raise the heat of the oven to 400°F and bake for another 15 minutes.
7. Lower the heat to 230°F and bake for another 45-60 minutes.
8. Turn off the heat and let the dessert cool in the oven. Remove it when it has cooled completely and place it in the fridge to rest overnight. Serve it with fresh blueberries.

Nutrition:

Calories: 158

Protein: 5 Grams

Fat: 8 Grams

Net Carbs: 21 Gram

Keto Gingerbread Crème Brule

Preparation Time: 15 minutes

Cooking Time: 30 minutes

Servings: 6

Ingredients:

- 1¾ cups heavy whipping cream
- 2 tsp pumpkin pie spice
- 2 tbsperythritol (an all-natural sweetener)
- ¼ tsp vanilla extract
- 4 egg yolks
- ½ clementine (optional)

Directions:

1. Preheat the oven to 360°F.
2. Crack the eggs to separate them and place the egg whites and the egg yolks in two separate bowls. We will only use egg yolks in this recipe, so save the egg whites for a rainy day.
3. Add some cream to a saucepan and bring it to a boil along with the spices, vanilla extract, and sweetener mixed in.
4. Add the warm cream mixture into the egg yolks. Do this slowly, only adding a little bit at a time, while whisking.
5. Pour it into oven-proof ramekins or small Pyrex bowls that are firmly placed in a larger baking dish with large sides.
6. Add some water to the larger dish with the ramekins in it until it's about halfway up the ramekins. Make sure not to get water in the ramekins though. The water helps the cream cook gently and evenly for a creamy and smooth result.
7. Bake it in the oven for about 30 minutes. Take the ramekins out from

the baking dish and let the dessert cool.

8. You can enjoy this dessert either warm or cold, you can also add a clementine segment on top of it.

Nutrition:

Calories: 321

Protein: 14 Grams

Fat: 1 Grams

Net Carbs: 11 Gram

Tuscan Chicken

Preparation Time: 10 minutes

Cooking Time: 30 minutes

Servings: 2

Ingredients:

- 1 lb. boneless and skinless chicken thighs
- 3 tbsps. olive oil
- 6 green onions, chopped
- 1 1/2 cups white wine
- 1 1/2 cups chicken broth
- 1 branch of fresh rosemary
- 1/3 cup black and green olives, pitted and roughly chopped
- Salt and pepper

Directions:

1. In a large skillet, brown the chicken in the oil. Salt lightly (be careful, the olives are already salted) and pepper.
2. Add green onions and continue cooking for about 2 minutes. Add half of the white wine and simmer until evaporated.
3. Add half of the broth, rosemary, and olives. Simmer on low heat until the liquid has reduced by half.

4. Add the remaining wine and broth gradually during cooking as soon as the liquid has reduced by half (see note). Return the chicken a few times during cooking to coat it well in the sauce.
5. Simmer over low heat for about 30 minutes, until the chicken becomes fluffy; check that with a fork and check if the sauce has thickened.
6. Adjust seasoning. Remove the rosemary branch.
7. Divide the chicken thighs between 2 containers
8. Lock the containers and store your dinner in the refrigerator
9. Storage, freeze, thaw and reheat guideline:
10. This Tuscan Chicken can be stored in the refrigerator at 40 °F in a plastic container for about 2 days. When you want to consume your dinner, remove the chicken from the refrigerator and microwave it for about 5 minutes.

Nutrition:

Calories: 505

Fat: 42 g

Carbs: 5.8 g

Protein 26 g

Sugar: 1 g;

Steak with Broccoli

Preparation Time: 5 minutes

Cooking Time: 5 minutes

Servings: 3

Ingredients:

- 1/2 small thinly sliced red onion
- 3 tbsp of red wine vinegar
- 1 pinch of kosher salt

- 1 Pinch of freshly ground black pepper
- 5 tbsp of divided extra-virgin olive oil
- 1 and 1/4 lb. of cut skirt steak
- 1 tsp of ground coriander
- 1 thinly sliced small head of broccoli
- 4 c. of Mache
- 1/4 Cup roasted sunflower seeds
- 4 oz., 1/4 cup shaved ricotta

Directions:

1. Combine the vinegar and about 1/2 tsp. salt in a bowl. Then set it aside
2. Meanwhile, press the function sauté of your Instant pot and heat about 1 tbsp. in it; then season the steak with the coriander, the salt, and the pepper.
3. Lock the lid of your Instant Pot
4. Cook for about 5 minutes at a temperature of 365°F
5. Add the broccoli, the Mache, the sunflower seeds, and the remaining 4 tbsps. oil to the onions and toss to combine it.
6. Season the steak with 1 pinch of salt and the pepper.
7. Storage, freeze, thaw and reheat guideline:
8. To store your dinner, divide it between 3 containers; then put the containers in the refrigerator at a temperature of about 40°F. When you are ready to serve your dinner, remove the containers from the refrigerator and microwave it for about 4 minutes

Nutrition:

Calories: 460

Fat: 37.6g

Carbs: 8.5 g

Protein 21.7g

Sugar: 2.3g

Instant Pot Ketogenic Chili

Preparation Time: 5 minutes

Cooking Time: 30 minutes

Servings: 2

Ingredients:

- 1 lb. of ground Beef
- 1 lb. of ground Sausage
- 1 Medium, chopped green Bell Pepper
- 1/2 Medium, chopped yellow onion
- 1 can of 6 oz. of tomato paste
- 2 tbsps. olive oil
- 1 tbsp. avocado oil
- 1 Tbsp of chili Powder
- ½ Tbsp of ground Cumin
- 3 to 4 minced garlic cloves
- 1/3 to ½ cup water
- 1 can of 14.05 diced tomatoes in the tomato Juice

Directions:

1. Preheat your Instant pot by pressing the "Sauté" button
2. Add in the olive oil and avocado oil; then add the ground beef and the sausage to the Instant pot and cook until it becomes brown.
3. Once the meat is browned set the Instant Pot to the function "keep warm/cancel."
4. Add in the rest of the **Ingredients:** into your Instant Pot and mix very well.
5. Cover the lid of the instant pot and lock it; then make sure that the steam valve is sealed
6. Select the function Bean/Chilli setting for around 30 minutes
7. Once the chili is perfectly cooked, the Instant Pot will automatically shift to the function mode "Keep Warm

8. Let the pressure release naturally, or you can rather use the quick release method.

9. Divide the chili between 2 containers; then top with chopped parsley

10. Store the containers in the refrigerator for two days

Nutrition:

Calories: 555

Fat: 46.5g

Carbs: 9.1 g

Protein 24.9g

Sugar: 3g

Ahi Tuna Bowl

Preparation Time: 10 minutes

Cooking Time: 5 minutes

Servings: 2

Ingredients:

- 1 lb. of diced ahi tuna, chopped
- 1 tbsp of coconut Aminos
- ½ tsp of sesame oil
- 1/4 cup mayonnaise
- 2 tbsps. cream cheese
- 2 Tbsps. sriracha
- 1 Diced, ripe avocado
- 1/2 cup Kimchi
- ½ Cup chopped green onion
- 1 tbsp. avocado oil
- 1 pinch of sesame seeds

Directions:

1. Add the avocado oil to the bowl; then add the diced tuna.

2. Add the coconut aminos, the cream cheese, the sesame oil, the mayo, the sriracha to the

bowl and toss it very well to combine.

3. Add the diced avocado and the kimchi to the bowl and combine it very well.

4. Divide the Kimchi between two containers; then add the greens, the cauliflower rice and the chopped green onion with the sesame seeds

5. Store the containers in the refrigerator for 2 days.

Nutrition:

Calories: 345

Fat: 26.5 g

Carbs: 6.6 g

Protein 19.8 g

Sugar: 1.4g

Stuffed Spinach and Beef Burgers

Preparation Time: 5 minutes

Cooking Time: 8 minutes

Servings: 2

Ingredients:

- 1 lb. of ground chuck roast
- 1 tsp. salt
- ¾ tsp. ground black pepper
- 2 tbsps. cream cheese
- 1 tbsp. avocado oil
- 1 cup firmly packed fresh spinach
- ½ cup shredded mozzarella cheese (4 to 5 oz.)
- 2 tbsps. grated Parmesan cheese

Directions:

1. In a large bowl, combine the ground beef with the salt, and the pepper.

2. Scoop about 1/3 cup the mixture and with wet hands; shape about 4 patties about ½-inch of thickness. Place the patties in the refrigerator.
3. Place the spinach in a saucepan over medium-high heat.
4. Cover the pan and cook for about 2 minutes, until the spinach becomes wilted.
5. Drain the spinach and let cool; then squeeze the spinach
6. Cut the spinach and put it in a bowl; then stir in the mozzarella cheese, the cream cheese, the avocado oil, and the Parmesan.
7. Scoop ¼ cup the stuffing and shape 4 patties; then cover with the remaining 4 patties
8. Seal both the edges of each burger
9. Cup each of the patties with your hands to make it round
10. Press each of the patties a little bit to make a thick layer Heat your grilling pan over a high heat
11. Grill your burgers for about 6 minutes on each of the two sides.
12. Divide the burgers between 2 containers
13. Store in the refrigerator Serve!

Nutrition:
Calories: 450 Fat: 37 g
Carbs: 7 g Protein 22 g
Sugar: 1.9g

Ketogenic Low Carb Cloud Bread
Preparation Time: 10 minutes
Cooking Time: 15 minutes
Servings: 3
Ingredients:

- 1 tsp. baking powder

- 1 Cup Philadelphia cheese
- 3 Organic egg

Directions:
1. Separate the whites from the yolks of the three eggs. Place the whites in one bowl and the yolks in the other.
2. Add the cheese at room temperature to the yolks and mix with an electric mixer to obtain a fine paste.
3. Add the baking soda to the egg whites and mix with the mixer.
4. Mix both mixtures gently with a spatula.
5. Preheat the oven to 300°F. Spread small circles of dough on parchment paper
6. , cook for 15 to 20 minutes.
7. Once the cloud bread is cooked, set it aside to cool for about 5 minutes
8. Divide the cloud bread between 3 plastic wraps; then plastic the plastic wraps in two containers
9. Store the containers in the refrigerator for 3 days

Nutrition:
Calories: 200 Fat: 17g
Carbs: 2 g Protein 10g Sugar: 3g

Ketogenic Bruschetta
Preparation Time: 10 minutes
Cooking Time: 45 minutes
Servings: 3
Ingredients:

- 1 tsp. baking powder

- 1 Cup Philadelphia cheese
- 3 Organic egg
- 1 and ½ cups black olives
- 1 caper
- 24 cherry tomatoes
- oregano
- olive oil
- 1 clove of garlic

Directions:

1. Wash, dry and put the peppers on a baking sheet covered with parchment paper.
2. Bake at 400° F for one hour, turning over on the other side after 30 minutes.
3. Put the roasted peppers in a food bag for 15 minutes.
4. Clean the peppers removing the skin and seeds.
5. Put the peppers on a plate and season with olive oil
6. Wash, dry and halve the cherry tomatoes.
7. Heat a peel and roast the tomatoes on both sides.
8. Toss the slices of Pan Bruschetta so that they are crunchy on the outside.
9. Rub the clove of garlic on the slices of bread.
10. Put the pitted olives in the bowl of a blender and mash them.
11. Coat the slices with olive puree, then cover with peppers cut in fillets, add the tomatoes, some capers, sprinkle with oregano and drizzle with a little olive oil

Nutrition:

Calories: 410 Fat: 35g

Carbs: 7.5 g Protein 16g

Sugar: 1g

Cauliflower Pizza

Preparation Time: 10 minutes

Cooking Time: 20 minutes

Servings: 2

Ingredients:

- 1 cauliflower
- ½ cup grated mozzarella
- 1 organic egg
- 1 cup white ham
- 1 cup mozzarella
- 4 tbsp of tomato sauce
- ½ cup grated cheese
- 1 tsp. oregano

Directions:

1. Cut the cauliflower head into small florets
2. Grate the cauliflower; the heat it for 4 minutes in the microwave
3. Fluff the cauliflower with a fork
4. Mix the egg and grated cheese with drained cauliflower until you obtain the dough
5. Spread the obtained mixture on a sheet of parchment paper and bake at 400°F until golden brown for about 15 to 20 minutes.
6. Garnish your pizza with olive and capers and
7. It's ready
8. Cut the pizza; then divide the portions between 2 containers and store it in the refrigerator for 2 days

Nutrition:

Calories: 430 Fat: 35.4g Carbs: 7 g

Protein 22.8g Sugar: 3g

Chicken Pizzaiola

Preparation Time: 10 minutes

Cooking Time: 20 minutes

Servings: 3

Ingredients:

- 3 chicken breasts
- 1 tray with ham
- 1 cup pasta sauce
- 1 and ½ cups grated cheese
- 1 Pinch of salt and pepper
- 2 Tbsps. olive oil

Directions:

1. Preheat the oven to 290 °F
2. Place the 3 chicken breasts on a sheet of parchment paper directly on the plate of your oven.
3. Slice the breasts partially and garnish with sauce, ham, and cheese.
4. Cover with grated cheese, season with salt and pepper and drizzle with oil.
5. Bake in a hot oven for 20 minutes
6. Once ready, divide the 2 chicken breasts between three containers
7. Seal the containers very well and store it in the refrigerator for 3 days

Nutrition:

Calories: 453

Fat: 34.8 g

Carbs: 8.9 g

Protein 26g

Sugar: 1.5 g

Beef Stroganoff with Protein Noodles

Preparation Time: 14 minutes

Cooking Time: 29 min

Servings: 1

Ingredients:

- 2 oz. Barilla Protein Farfalle Pasta
- ½ cup fresh sliced mushrooms
- 2 Tbls of chopped onion
- 1 T butter
- dash of black pepper
- 6 oz. steak, sliced thinly
- 1 T tomato paste
- ¼ tsp of Dijon mustard
- ½ cup beef broth
- ½ small container plain Greek yogurt

Directions:

1. Cook the pasta in water.
2. Place the butter in a Teflon skillet.
3. Next add in the onions, and mushrooms, cook until onions are shiny and water is gone.
4. Add the beef and brown well.
5. Stir in remaining ingredients except the pasta and yogurt.
6. Cook this until the beef is done, approximately 9 minutes.
7. Drain the pasta.
8. If the sauce is too thin, add 1 tsp low carb flax meal and boil to thicken.
9. Turn back down to low. Then add the yogurt to the sauce.

10. Serve the stroganoff over the pasta.

Nutrition:

Calories: 559

Total Fat: 23g;

Protein: 55g

Total Carbs: 4g

Dietary Fiber: 13g

Sugar: 2g

Sodium: 957mg

Beefy Tostadas

Preparation Time: 4 minute

Cooking Time: 9 minutes

Servings: 2

Ingredients:

- ¼ pound ground sirloin
- ¼ cup onions, minced
- 1 tsp garlic, minced
- 1 T olive oil
- ½ cup chopped green, red, and yellow peppers
- ½ cup cheddar cheese, mild or sharp, hand-shredded
- 2 Tortilla factory low-carb tortillas
- 2 T butter
- 1 c Greek yogurt, plain
- 2 T salsa verde

Directions:

1. Brown the tortillas in the butter. Place on a warm plate.
2. Cook the sirloin, onions, garlic, peppers in the olive oil.
3. Place on the tortillas.
4. Top with the cheese.
5. Add the Greek yogurt.
6. Drizzle with the salsa.

Nutrition:

Calories: 735

Total Fat: 48g

Protein: 66g

Total Carbs: 18g

Dietary Fiber: 8g

Sugar: 0g

Sodium: 708mg

Bratwurst German Dinner

Preparation Time: 4 minutes

Cooking Time: 19 minutes

Servings:

Ingredients:

- 1 Bratwurst sausage
- ½ cup sliced onion
- ½ cup sauerkraut, this includes the liquid
- 1 tsp olive oil
- Sprinkle of black pepper

Directions:

1. Cook the bratwurst and the onion in the olive oil, in a coated skillet.
2. Remove the bratwurst to a plate.
3. Place the sauerkraut into the skillet and cook 3 min.
4. Add the bratwurst and onion back to warm and mingle the flavors.
5. Sprinkle with black pepper and serve.

Nutrition:

Calories: 332 Total Fat: 26g

Protein: 15g Total Carbs: 8g

Dietary Fiber: 9g Sugar: 4g

Sodium: 1188mg

Cajun Blackened Fish with Cauliflower Salad

Preparation Time: 9 minutes
Cooking Time: 9 minutes
Servings: 1
Ingredients:

- 1 cup chopped cauliflower
- 1 tsp red pepper flakes
- 1 T Italian seasonings
- 1 T garlic, minced
- 6 oz. tilapia
- 1 cup English cucumber, chopped with peel
- 2 T olive oil
- 1 sprig dill, chopped
- 1 Sweetener packet
- 3 T lime juice
- 2 T Cajun blackened seasoning

Directions:

1. Mix the seasonings, except the Cajun blackened seasoning, into one bowl.
2. Add 1 T olive oil.
3. Emulsify or whip.
4. Pour the dressing over the cauliflower and cucumber.
5. Brush the fish with the olive oil on both sides.
6. Pour the other 1 T oil into a coated skillet.
7. Press the Cajun seasoning onto both sides of the fish.
8. Cook the fish in the olive oil 3 minutes per side.
9. Plate and serve.

Nutrition:
Calories: 530
Total Fat: 33.5g
Protein: 32g
Total Carbs: 5.5g
Dietary Fiber: 4g
Sugar: 3g
Sodium: 80mg

Chicken Parmesan over Protein Pasta

Preparation Time: 9 minutes
Cooking Time: 14 minutes
Servings: 2
Ingredients:

- 1 dash black pepper
- ½ tsp Italian spice mix
- 8 oz. Protein Plus Spaghetti
- ½ hand-shredded Parmesan
- 1 diced zucchini squash
- 1 ½ cups marinara sauce, any brand
- 24 oz. boneless thin chicken cutlets
- 2 T olive oil
- ½ cup grated Mozzarella cheese
- Water, for boiling the pasta

Directions:

1. Boil the pasta with the zucchini in the water.
2. Mix the Italian spices and ¼ cup Parmesan cheese and place in a shallow dish.
3. Brush the chicken pieces with olive oil and press into spice and cheese to coat.
4. Place in skillet with the oil and cook until done.

5. Add the marinara sauce to the skillet to warm, cover the chicken if you desire.
6. Drain the pasta and zucchini, place on plates.
7. Top the chicken with the mozzarella and remaining Parmesan cheese.
8. Place sauce, chicken, and cheese onto spaghetti and serve.

Nutrition:

Calories: 372 Total Fat: 18g

Protein: 56g Total Carbs: 7 g

Dietary Fiber: 2g

Sugar: 6g

Sodium: 1335mg

Chicken Chow Mein Stir Fry

Preparation Time: 9 minutes

Cooking Time: 14 minutes

Servings: 4

Ingredients:

- 1/2 cup sliced onion
- 2 T Oil, sesame garlic flavored
- 4 cups shredded Bok-Choy
- 1 c Sugar Snap Peas
- 1 cup fresh bean sprouts
- 3 stalks Celery, chopped
- 1 1/2 tsp minced Garlic
- 1 packet Splenda
- 1 cup Broth, chicken
- 2 T Soy Sauce
- 1 T ginger, freshly minced
- 1 tsp cornstarch
- 4 boneless Chicken Breasts, cooked/sliced thinly

Directions:

1. Place the bok-choy, peas, celery in a skillet with 1 T garlic oil.
2. Stir fry until bok-choy is softened to liking.
3. Add remaining ingredients except the cornstarch.
4. If too thin, stir cornstarch into ½ cup cold water. When smooth pour into skillet.
5. Bring cornstarch and chow mein to a one-minute boil. Turn off the heat source.
6. Stir sauce then for wait 4 minutes to serve, after the chow mein has thickened.

Nutrition:

Calories: 368

Total Fat: 18g

Protein: 42g

Total Carbs: 12g

Dietary Fiber: 16g

Sugar: 6g

Sodium: 746mg

Colorful Chicken Casserole

Preparation Time: 14 minutes

Cooking Time: 14 minutes

Servings: 6

Ingredients:

- 1 cup broth, chicken
- 3 cups cooked chicken, diced
- 4 cups chopped broccoli
- 1 cup assorted colored bell peppers, chopped
- 1 cup cream
- 4 T sherry

- ¼ c hand-shredded Parmesan cheese
- 1 small size can black olives, sliced, drained
- 2 Tortilla Factory low-carb whole wheat tortillas
- ½ c hand-shredded mozzarella

Directions:

1. Place broccoli and chicken broth into a skillet.
2. Top with lid, bring to a boil, and steam until desired crispness. (4 min)
3. Add the peppers, steam for one minute if you don't want them crisp.
4. Add the chicken and stir to heat.
5. Combine the sherry, cream, parmesan, and olives.
6. Tear the tortillas into bite-sized pieces.
7. Stir into the chicken and broccoli.
8. Pour cream sauce over the chicken, stir.
9. Top with hand-shredded mozzarella.
10. Broil in oven until cheese is melted and golden brown.

Nutrition:

Calories: 412

Total Fat: 30g

Protein: 29

Total Carbs: 10g

Dietary Fiber: 9g

Sugar: 1g

Sodium: 712mg

Chicken Relleno Casserole

Preparation Time: 19 minutes

Cooking Time: 29 minutes

Servings: 6

Ingredients:

- 6 Tortilla Factory low-carb whole wheat tortillas, torn into small pieces
- 1 ½ cups hand-shredded cheese, Mexican
- 1 beaten egg
- 1 cup milk
- 2 cups cooked chicken, shredded
- 1 can Ro-tel
- ½ cup salsa verde

Directions:

1. Grease an 8 x 8 glass baking dish
2. Heat oven to 375 degrees
3. Combine everything together, but reserve ½ cup of the cheese
4. Bake it for 29 minutes
5. Take it out of oven and add ½ cup cheese
6. Broil for about 2 minutes to melt the cheese

Nutrition:

Calories: 265

Total Fat: 16g

Protein: 20g

Total Carbs: 18g

Dietary Fiber: 10g

Sugar: 0g

Sodium: 708mg

CHAPTER 4:

Soup and Stew

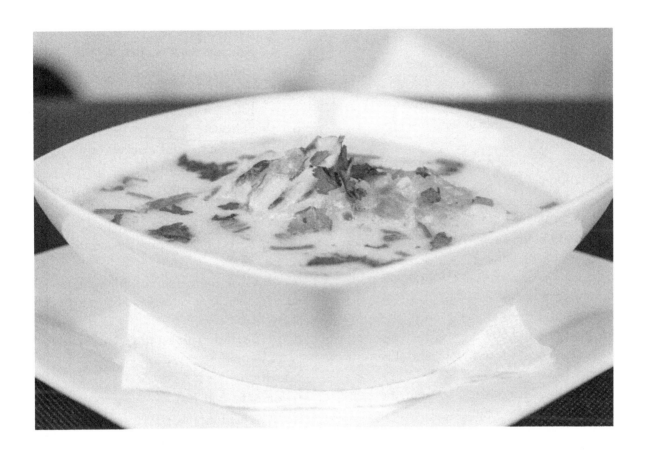

Cheesy Cauliflower Soup

Preparation Time: 10 minutes

Cooking Time: 30 minutes

Servings: 8

Ingredients:

- ¼ cup butter
- 1 head cauliflower, chopped
- ½ onion, chopped
- ½ teaspoon ground nutmeg
- 4 cups chicken stock
- 1 cup heavy whipping cream
- Salt and freshly ground black pepper, to taste
- 1 cup Cheddar cheese, shredded

Directions:

1. Take a large stockpot and place it over medium heat.
2. Add butter to this pot and let it melt.
3. Add cauliflower and onion to the melted butter and sauté for 10 minutes until these veggies are soft.
4. Add nutmeg and chicken stock to the pot and bring to a boil.
5. Reduce the heat to low and allow it to simmer for 15 minutes.
6. Remove the stockpot from the heat and then add heavy cream.
7. Purée the cooked soup with an immersion blender until smooth.
8. Sprinkle this soup with salt and black pepper.
9. Garnish with Cheddar cheese and serve warm.

Nutrition:

Calories: 224 Fat: 16.8g

Total carbs: 10.8g Fiber: 2.2g

Protein: 9.6g

Egg Broth

Preparation Time: 5 minutes

Cooking Time: 5 minutes

Servings: 4

Ingredients:

- 2 tablespoons unsalted butter
- 4 cups chicken broth
- 3 large eggs
- Salt and black pepper, to taste
- 1 sliced green onion, for garnish

Directions:

1. Take a medium stockpot and place it over high heat.
2. Add butter and chicken broth to the pot and bring to a boil.
3. Break eggs into a bowl and beat them for 1 minute with a fork until frothy.
4. Once the broth boils, slowly pour in beaten eggs while stirring the broth with a spoon.
5. Cook for 1 minute with continuously stirring, then sprinkle salt and black pepper to season.
6. Garnish with sliced green onion, then serve warm.

Nutrition:

Calories: 93 Fat: 7.8g

Total carbs: 1.8g Fiber: 0.1g

Protein: 3.9g

Cauliflower Cream Soup

Preparation Time: 15 minutes

Cooking Time: 4 hours 10 minutes

Servings: 5

Ingredients:

- 10 slices bacon

- 3 small heads cauliflower, cored and cut into florets
- 4 cups chicken broth
- ¼ cup (½ stick) salted butter
- 3 cloves garlic, pressed
- ½ large yellow onion, chopped
- 1 cup heavy whipping cream
- 2 cups Cheddar cheese, shredded
- Salt and black pepper, to taste
- Freshly chopped chives or green onions, for garnish

Directions:

1. Take a large skillet and place it over medium heat.

2. Add bacon to the skillet and cook for about 8 minutes until brown and crispy.

3. Transfer the cooked bacon to a paper towel-lined plate to absorb the excess grease.

4. Allow the bacon to cool, then chop it. Wrap the plate of chopped bacon in plastic and refrigerate it.

5. Add the cauliflower florets to the food processor and pulse until chopped thoroughly.

6. Add chicken broth, butter, garlic, onion, and chopped cauliflower to the slow cooker.

7. Give all these ingredients a gentle stir, then put on the lid.

8. Cook the cauliflower soup for 4 hours on high heat.

9. Once the cauliflower is tender, purée the soup with an immersion blender until smooth.

10. Add chopped bacon, heavy cream, cheese, salt, and black pepper. Mix well and let the cheese melt in the hot soup.

11. Garnish with green onions or chives, then serve warm.

Nutrition:
Calories: 627
Fat: 54.3g
Total carbs: 13.7g
Fiber: 3.7g
Protein: 24.6g

Shrimp Mushroom Chowder

Preparation Time: 10 minutes
Cooking Time: 40 minutes
Servings: 6
Ingredients:

- ¼ cup refined avocado oil
- 1/3 cup diced yellow onions
- 1 2/3 cups diced mushrooms
- 10½ ounces (298 g) small raw shrimp, shelled and deveined
- 1 can (131/2-ounce / 383-g) unsweetened coconut milk
- 1/3 cup chicken bone broth
- 2 tablespoons apple cider vinegar
- 1 teaspoon onion powder
- 1 teaspoon paprika
- 1 bay leaf
- ¾ teaspoon finely ground gray sea salt
- ½ teaspoon dried oregano leaves
- ¼ teaspoon ground black pepper
- 1 medium zucchini (7-ounce / 198-g), cubed
- 12 radishes (6-ounce / 170-g), cubed

Directions:

1. Add avocado oil to a large saucepan and place it over medium heat.

2. Add onions and mushrooms to the pan and sauté for 10 minutes or until onions are soft and mushrooms are lightly browned.

3. Stir in shrimp, coconut milk, chicken broth, apple cider vinegar, onion powder, paprika, bay leaf, sea salt, oregano leaves, and black pepper.

4. Cover the soup mixture with a lid and cook for 20 minutes on low heat.

5. Add zucchini and radishes to the soup and cook for 10 minutes.

6. Remove the bay leaf from the soup and divide the soup into 6 small serving bowls. Serve hot.

Nutrition:

Calories: 311 Fat: 26.3g

Total carbs: 7.7g Fiber: 2.9g

Protein: 13.7g

Pork Tarragon Soup

Preparation Time: 10 minutes

Cooking Time: 1 hour 20 minutes

Servings: 6

Ingredients:

- 1/3 cup lard
- 1 pound (454 g) pork loin, cut into ½-inch (1.25-cm) pieces
- 10 strips bacon (about 10-ounce / 284-g), cut into ½-inch (1.25-cm) pieces
- ¾ cup sliced shallots
- 3 medium turnips (about 12½-ounce / 354-g), cubed
- 1 tablespoon yellow mustard
- ¼ cup dry white wine
- 1¾ cups chicken bone broth
- 4 sprigs fresh thyme
- 2 tablespoons unflavored gelatin
- 2 tablespoons apple cider vinegar
- ½ cup unsweetened coconut milk
- 1 tablespoon dried tarragon leaves

Directions:

1. Take a large saucepan and place it over medium heat.

2. Add lard to the saucepan and allow it to melt.

3. Add pork pieces to the melted lard and sauté for 8 minutes until golden brown.

4. Add bacon pieces and sliced shallots and sauté for 5 minutes or until fragrant.

5. Add turnips, mustard, wine, bone broth, and thyme sprigs to the soup.

6. Mix these ingredients gently and cover this soup with a lid.

7. Bring the soup to a boil, then reduce the heat to medium-low. Cook this soup for 1 hour.

8. Remove and discard the thyme sprigs from the soup then add gelatin, vinegar, coconut milk, and tarragon.

9. Increase the heat to medium and bring the soup to a boil. Cover to cook for 10 minutes.

10. Divide the cooked soup into 6 serving bowls and serve warm.

Nutrition:

Calories: 566 Fat: 41.5g

Total carbs: 9.7g Fiber: 1.2g Protein: 39.6g

Creamy Broccoli and Cauliflower Soup

Preparation Time: 20 minutes

Cooking Time: 15 minutes

Servings: 6

Ingredients:

- 1 (13½-ounce / 383-g) can unsweetened coconut milk
- 2 cups vegetable stock

- 1 (14-ounce / 397-g) small head cauliflower, cored and cut into large florets
- 2 medium celery sticks, chopped
- 1 teaspoon finely ground gray sea salt
- 6 green onions, green parts only, roughly chopped
- 1 large head broccoli, cored and cut into large florets
- ¼ teaspoon ground black pepper
- ¼ teaspoon ground white pepper
- 1/3 cup butter-infused olive oil
- 1 chopped green onion, for garnish

Directions:

1. Take a large saucepan and place it over medium heat.

2. Add coconut milk, vegetable stock, cauliflower florets, chopped celery, salt, and green onions.

3. Mix them gently, then cover and bring the soup to a boil.

4. Continue cooking the soup for 15 minutes until the cauliflower florets are soft.

5. Meanwhile, blanch the broccoli in a pot of boiling water for 1 minute until soft but still crisp, then drain on a paper towel. Set aside on a plate.

6. When the cauliflower soup is cooked, transfer it to a blender.

7. Add black pepper, white pepper, and olive oil. Blend the soup for 1 minute until smooth.

8. Add the soft broccoli and blend again for 30 seconds.

9. Divide the cooked broccoli and cauliflower soup into 6 serving bowls.

10. Garnish with chopped green onions and serve warm.

Nutrition:

Calories: 264 Fat: 23.3g
Total carbs: 10.3g Fiber: 3.6g
Protein: 6.9g

Chicken Turnip Soup

Preparation Time: 10 minutes
Cooking Time: 6 to 8 hours
Servings: 5
Ingredients:

- 12 ounces (340g) bone-in chicken
- ¼ cup turnip, chopped
- ¼ cup onions, chopped
- 4 garlic cloves, smashed
- 4 cups water
- 3 sprigs thyme
- 2 bay leaves
- Salt, to taste
- ¼ teaspoon freshly ground black pepper

Directions:

1. Put the chicken, turnip, onions, garlic, water, thyme springs, and bay leaves in a slow cooker.

2. Season with salt and pepper, then give the mixture a good stir.

3. Cover and cook on low for 6 to 8 hours until the chicken is cooked through.

4. When ready, remove the bay leaves and shred the chicken with a fork.

5. Divide the soup among five bowls and serve.

Nutrition:

Calories: 186 Fat: 13.6g
Total carbs: 3.3g Fiber: 2.6g
Protein: 15.2g

Spinach Mushroom Soup

Preparation Time: 10 minutes

Cooking Time: 5 minutes

Servings: 3

Ingredients:

- 1 tablespoon olive oil
- 1 teaspoon garlic, finely chopped
- 1 cup spinach, torn into small pieces
- ½ cup mushrooms, chopped
- Salt and freshly ground black pepper, to taste
- ½ teaspoon tamari
- 3 cups vegetable stock
- 1 teaspoon sesame seeds, roasted

Directions:

1. Place a saucepan over medium heat and add olive oil to heat.
2. Add garlic to the hot oil and sauté for 30 seconds or until fragrant.
3. Add spinach and mushrooms, then sauté for 1 minute or until lightly tender.
4. Add salt, black pepper, tamari, and vegetable stock. Cook for another 3 minutes. Stir constantly.
5. Garnish with sesame seeds and serve warm.

Nutrition:

Calories: 80 Fat: 7.4g Total carbs: 3.2g Fiber: 1.1g Protein: 1.2g

Garlicky Chicken Soup

Preparation Time: 10 minutes

Cooking Time: 10 minutes

Servings: 4

Ingredients:

- 2 tablespoons butter
- 1 large chicken breast cut into strips
- 4 ounces (113 g) cream cheese, cubed
- 2 tablespoons Garlic Gusto Seasoning
- ½ cup heavy cream
- 14½ ounces (411 g) chicken broth
- Salt, to taste

Directions:

1. Place a saucepan over medium heat and add butter to melt.
2. Add chicken strips and sauté for 2 minutes.
3. Add cream cheese and seasoning, and cook for 3 minutes, stirring occasionally.
4. Pour in the heavy cream and chicken broth. Bring the soup to a boil, then lower the heat.
5. Allow the soup to simmer for 4 minutes, then sprinkle with salt.
6. Let cool for 5 minutes and serve while warm.

Nutrition:

Calories: 243

Fat: 22.5g

Total carbs: 7.0g

Fiber: 6.6g

Protein: 9.6g

Cauliflower Curry Soup

Preparation Time: 15 minutes

Cooking Time: 26 minutes

Servings: 4

Ingredients:

- 2 tablespoons avocado oil
- 1 white onion, chopped
- 4 garlic cloves, chopped
- ½ Serrano pepper, seeds removed and chopped
- 1-inch ginger, chopped

- ¼ teaspoon turmeric powder
- 2 teaspoons curry powder
- ½ teaspoon black pepper
- 1 teaspoon salt
- 1 cup of water
- 1 large cauliflower, cut into florets
- 1 cup chicken broth
- 1 can unsweetened coconut milk
- Cilantro, for garnish

Directions:

1. Place a saucepan over medium heat and add oil to heat.

2. Add onions to the hot oil and sauté them for 3 minutes.

3. Add garlic, Serrano pepper, and ginger, then sauté for 2 minutes.

4. Add turmeric, curry powder, black pepper, and salt. Cook for 1 minute after a gentle stir.

5. Pour water into the pan, then add cauliflower.

6. Cover this soup with a lid and cook for 10 minutes. Stir constantly.

7. Remove the soup from the heat and allow it to cool at room temperature.

8. Transfer this soup to a blender and purée the soup until smooth.

9. Return the soup to the saucepan and add broth and coconut milk. Cook for 10 minutes more and stir frequently.

10. Divide the soup into four bowls and sprinkle the cilantro on top for garnish before serving.

Nutrition:

Calories: 342

Fat: 29.1g

Total carbs: 18.3g

Fiber: 5.5g

Protein: 7.17g

Asparagus Cream Soup

Preparation Time: 15 minutes

Cooking Time: 22 minutes

Servings: 6

Ingredients:

- 4 tablespoons butter
- 1 small onion, chopped
- 6 cups low-sodium chicken broth
- Salt and black pepper, to taste
- 2 pounds (907g) asparagus, cut in half
- ½ cup sour cream

Directions:

1. Place a large pot over low heat and add butter to melt.

2. Add onion to the melted butter and sauté for 2 minutes or until soft.

3. Add chicken broth, salt, black pepper, and asparagus.

4. Bring the soup to a boil, then cover the lid and cook for 20 minutes.

5. Remove the pot from the heat and allow it to cool for 5 minutes.

6. Transfer the soup to a blender and blend until smooth.

7. Add sour cream and pulse again to mix well.

8. Serve fresh and warm.

Nutrition:

Calories: 138

Fat: 10.5g

Total carbs: 10.2g

Fiber: 3.5g

Protein: 5.9g

Red Gazpacho Cream Soup

Preparation Time: 15 minutes

Cooking Time: 20 minutes

Servings: 10

Ingredients:

- 1 large red bell pepper, halved
- 1 large green bell pepper, halved
- 2 tablespoons basil, freshly chopped
- 4 medium tomatoes
- 1 small red onion
- 1 large cucumber, diced
- 2 medium spring onions, diced
- 2 tablespoons apple cider vinegar
- 2 garlic cloves
- 2 tablespoons fresh lemon juice
- 1 cup extra virgin olive oil
- Salt and black pepper, to taste
- 1¼ pounds (567 g) feta cheese, shredded

Directions:

1. Preheat the oven to 400°F (205°C) and line a baking tray with parchment paper.

2. Place all the bell peppers in the baking tray and roast in the preheated oven for 20 minutes.

3. Remove the bell peppers from the oven. Allow to cool, then peel off their skin.

4. Transfer the peeled bell peppers to a blender along with basil, tomatoes, red onions, cucumber, spring onions, vinegar, garlic, lemon juice, olive oil, black pepper, and salt. Blend until the mixture smooth.

5. Add black pepper and salt to taste.

6. Garnish with feta cheese and serve warm.

Nutrition:

Calories: 248 Fat: 21.6g Total carbs: 8.3g Fiber: 4.1g Protein: 9.3g

Beef Taco Soup

Preparation Time: 15 minutes

Cooking Time: 24 minutes

Servings: 8

Ingredients:

- 2 garlic cloves, minced
- ½ cup onions, chopped
- 1 pound (454 g) ground beef
- 1 teaspoon chili powder
- 1 tablespoon ground cumin
- 1 (8-ounce / 227-g) package cream cheese, softened
- 2 (10-ounce / 284-g) cans diced tomatoes and green chilies
- ½ cup heavy cream
- 2 teaspoons salt
- 2 (14½-ounce / 411-g) cans beef broth

Directions:

1. Take a large saucepan and place it over medium-high heat.

2. Add garlic, onions, and ground beef to the soup and sauté for 7 minutes until beef is browned.

3. Add chili powder and cumin, then cook for 2 minutes.

4. Add cream cheese and cook for 5 minutes while mashing the cream cheese into the beef with a spoon.

5. Add diced tomatoes and green chilies, heavy cream, salt and broth then cook for 10 minutes.

6. Mix gently and serve warm.

Nutrition:

Calories: 205 Fat: 13.3g

Total carbs: 4.4g Fiber: 0.8g

Protein: 8.0g

Creamy Tomato Soup

Preparation Time: 15 minutes

Cooking Time: 30 minutes

Servings: 4

Ingredients:

- 2 cups of water
- 4 cups tomato juice
- 3 tomatoes, peeled, seeded and diced
- 14 leaves fresh basil
- 2 tablespoons butter
- 1 cup heavy whipping cream
- Salt and black pepper, to taste

Directions:

1. Take a suitable cooking pot and place it over medium heat.
2. Add water, tomato juice, and tomatoes, then simmer for 30 minutes.
3. Transfer the soup to a blender, then add basil leaves.
4. Press the pulse button and blend the soup until smooth.
5. Return this tomato soup to the cooking pot and place it over medium heat.
6. Add butter, heavy cream, salt, and black pepper. Cook and mix until the butter melts.
7. Serve warm and fresh.

Nutrition:

Calories: 203

Fat: 17.7g

Total carbs: 13.0g

Fiber: 5.6g

Protein: 3.7g

Creamy Broccoli and Leek Soup

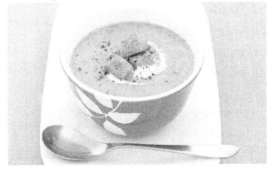

Preparation Time: 5 minutes

Cooking Time: 25 minutes

Servings: 4

Ingredients: 10 oz. broccoli

- 1 leek
- 8 oz. cream cheese
- 3 oz. butter
- 3 cups water
- 1 garlic clove
- ½ cup fresh basil
- salt and pepper

Directions:

1. Rinse the leek and chop both parts finely. Slice the broccoli thinly.
2. Place the veggies in a pot and cover with water and then season them. Boil the water until the broccoli softens.
3. Add the florets and garlic, while lowering the heat.
4. Add in the cheese, butter, pepper, and basil. Blend until desired consistency: if too thick use water; if you want to make it thicker, use a little bit of heavy cream.

Nutrition:

Calories: 451 kcal Fats: 37 g Protein: 10 g

Carbs: 4 g

Chicken Soup

Preparation Time: 25 minutes
Cooking Time: 80 minutes
Servings: 4
Ingredients:

- 6 cups water
- 1 chicken
- 1 medium carrot
- 1 yellow onion
- 1 bay leaf
- 1 leek
- 2 garlic cloves
- 1 tbsp. dried thyme
- ½ cup white wine, dry (no, not for drinking)
- 1 tsp. peppercorns
- salt and pepper

Directions:

1. Peel and cut your veggies. Brown them in oil in a big pot.
2. Split your chicken in half, down on the middle. Pour water and spices in the pot. Let it simmer for one hour.
3. Take out the chicken save the meat, and toss away the bones.
4. Put the meat back in the pot, and let it simmer on medium heat for 20-25 minutes again, while seasoning to your liking.

Nutrition:

Calories: 145 kcal
Fats: 12 g
Carbs: 1 g
Protein: 8 g

Greek Egg and Lemon Soup with Chicken

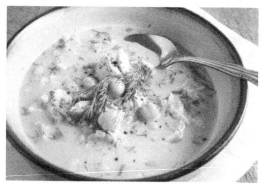

Preparation Time: 5 minutes
Cooking Time: 30 minutes
Servings: 4
Ingredients:

- 4 cups water
- ¾ lbs. cauli
- 1 lb. boneless chicken thighs
- 1/3 lb. butter
- 4 eggs
- 1 lemon
- 2 tbsps. fresh parsley
- 1 bay leaf
- 2 chicken bouillon cubes
- salt and pepper

Directions:

1. Slice your chicken thinly and then place in a saucepan while adding cold water and the cubes and bay leaf. Let the meat simmer for 10 minutes before removing it and the bay leaf.
2. Grate your cauli and place it in a saucepan. Add butter and boil for a few minutes.
3. Beat your eggs and lemon juice in a bowl, while seasoning it.

4. Reduce the heat a bit and add the eggs, stirring continuously. Let simmer but don't boil.
5. Return the chicken.

Nutrition:
Calories: 582 kcal
Carbs: 4 g
Fats: 49 g
Protein: 31 g

Wild Mushroom Soup

Preparation Time: 10 minutes
Cooking Time: 30 minutes
Servings: 4
Ingredients:

- 6 oz. mix of portabella mushrooms, oyster mushrooms, and shiitake mushrooms
- 3 cups water
- 1 garlic clove
- 1 shallot
- 4 oz. butter
- 1 chicken bouillon cube
- ½ lb. celery root
- 1 tbsp. white wine vinegar
- 1 cup heavy whipping cream
- fresh parsley

Directions:

1. Clean, trim, and chop your mushrooms and celery. Do the same to your shallot and garlic.
2. Sauté your chopped veggies in butter over medium heat in a saucepan.

3. Add thyme, vinegar, chicken bouillon cube, and water as you bring to boil. Then let it simmer for 10-15 minutes.
4. Add cream to them with an immersion blender until your desired consistency. Serve with parsley on top.

Nutrition:
Calories: 481 kcal
Fats: 47 g
Protein: 7 g
Carbs: 9 g

Roasted Butternut Squash Soup

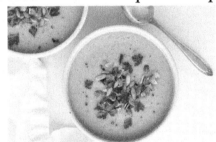

Preparation Time: 15 minutes
Cooking Time: 30 minutes
Servings: 4
Ingredients:

- 1 large butternut squash, cubed and peeled
- 1 stalk celery, sliced
- 2 potatoes, peeled, chopped
- 1 onion, chopped
- 1 large carrot, chopped
- 3 tbsps. olive oil
- 1 tbsp. fresh thyme
- 25 oz. chicken broth
- 1 tbsp. butter
- salt and pepper

Directions:

1. Preheat your oven to 400°F. On a baking sheet, toss squash and potatoes with 2 tbsp. oil and season to your taster. Roast for 20-25 minutes.
2. In the meantime, melt your butter and the rest of the oil in a large pot over medium heat. Add the onion, celery, carrot and cook for 5-8 minutes. Season them, too.
3. Add roasted squash and potatoes. Then pour over the chicken broth. Simmer it for 10 minutes using an immersion blender until the soup is creamy.
4. Garnish it with thyme.

Nutrition:

Calories: 254 kcal

Fats: 15 g

Carbs: 19 g

Protein: 6 g

Zucchini Cream Soup

Preparation Time: 5 minutes

Cooking Time: 20 minutes

Servings: 4

Ingredients:

- 3 zucchinis
- 32 oz. chicken broth
- 2 cloves garlic
- 2 tbsps. sour cream
- ½ small onion
- parmesan cheese (for topping if desired)

Directions:

1. Combine your broth, garlic, zucchini, and onion in a large pot over medium heat until boiling.
2. Lower the heat, cover, and let simmer for 15-20 minutes
3. Remove from heat and purée with an immersion blender, while adding the sour cream and pureeing until smooth.
4. Season to taste and top with your cheese.

Nutrition:

Calories: 117 kcal

Fats: 9 g

Carbs: 3 g

Protein: 4 g

Cauli Soup

Preparation Time: 5 minutes

Cooking Time: 25 minutes

Servings: 6

Ingredients:

- 32 oz. vegetable broth
- 1 head cauli, diced
- 2 garlic cloves, minced
- 1 onion, diced
- ½ tbsp. olive oil
- salt and pepper
- grated parmesan, sliced green onion for topping

Directions:

1. In a pot, heat oil over medium heat, while adding the onion and garlic. Then cook them for 4-5 minutes.

2. Add in the cauli and vegetable broth. Boil it and then cover for 15-20 minutes while covered.
3. Pour all contents of pot into a blender and season it.
4. Blend until smooth. Top it with your cheese and green onion.

Nutrition:

Calories: 37 kcal

Fats: 1 g

Carbs: 3 g

Protein: 3 g

Thai Coconut Soup

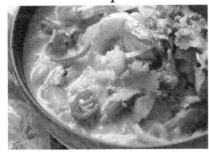

Preparation Time: 10 minutes

Cooking Time: 35 minutes

Servings: 4

Ingredients:

- 3 chicken breasts
- 9 oz. coconut milk
- 9 oz. chicken broth
- 2/3 tbsps. chili sauce
- 18 oz. water
- 2/3 tbsps. coconut aminos
- 2/3 oz. lime juice
- 2/3 tsps. ground ginger
- ¼ cup red boat fish sauce
- salt and pepper

Directions:

1. Slice up the chicken breasts thinly. Make them bite-sized.
2. In a large stock pot, mix your coconut milk, water, fish sauce, chili sauce, lime juice, ginger, coconut aminos, and broth. Bring to a boil.
3. Stir in chicken pieces. Then reduce the heat and cover pot, while simmering it for 30 minutes.
4. Remove the basil leaves and season it.

Nutrition:

Calories: 227 kcal Fats: 17 g

Carbs: 3 g Protein: 19 g

Chicken Ramen Soup

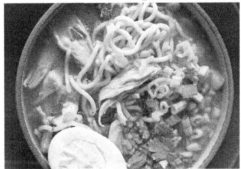

Preparation Time: 10 minutes

Cooking Time: 20 minutes

Servings: 2

Ingredients:

- 1 chicken breast
- 2 eggs
- 1 zucchini, made into noodles
- 4 cups chicken broth
- 2 cloves of garlic, peeled and minced

- 2 tbsps. coconut aminos
- 3 tbsps. avocado oil
- 1 tbsp. ginger

Directions:

1. Pan-fry the chicken in avocado oil in a pan until brown.
2. Hard boil your eggs and slice them in half.
3. Add chicken broth to a large pot and simmer with the garlic, coconut aminos, and ginger. Then add in the zucchini noodles for 4-5 minutes.
4. Put the broth into a bowl, top it with eggs and chicken slices, and season to your liking.

Nutrition:

Calories: 478 kcal Fats: 39 g

Carbs: 3 g Protein: 31 g

Chicken Broth and Egg Drop Soup

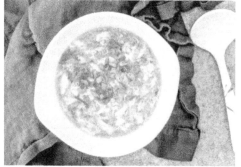

Preparation Time: 5 minutes

Cooking Time: 15 minutes

Servings: 2

Ingredients:

- 3 cups chicken broth
- 2 cups Swiss chard chopped

- 2 eggs, whisked
- 1 tsp. grated ginger
- 1 tsp. ground oregano
- 2 tbsps. coconut aminos
- salt and pepper

Directions:

1. Heat your broth in a saucepan.
2. Slowly drizzle in the eggs while stirring slowly.
3. Add the Swiss chard, grated ginger, oregano, and the coconut aminos. Next, season it and let it cook for 5-10 minutes.

Nutrition:

Calories: 225 kcal

Fats: 19 g

Carbs: 4 g

Protein: 11 g

Okra and Beef Stew

Preparation Time: 15 minutes

Cooking Time: 25 minutes

Servings: 3 servings

Ingredients:

- 6 oz. okra, chopped
- 8 oz. beef sirloin, chopped
- 1 cup of water
- ¼ cup coconut cream
- 1 teaspoon dried basil
- ¼ teaspoon cumin seeds
- 1 tablespoon avocado oil

Directions:

1. Sprinkle the beef sirloin with cumin seeds and dried basil and put in the instant pot.

2. Add avocado oil and roast the meat on saute mode for 5 minutes. Stir it occasionally.
3. Then add coconut cream, water, and okra.
4. Close the lid and cook the stew on manual mode (high pressure) for 25 minutes. Allow the natural pressure release for 10 minutes.

Nutrition:

Calories 216

Fat 10.2

Fiber 2.5

Carbs 5.7

Protein 24.6

Chipotle Stew

Preparation Time: 15 minutes

Cooking Time: 10 minutes

Servings: 3 servings

Ingredients:

- 2 chipotle chili in adobo sauce, chopped
- 1 oz. fresh cilantro, chopped
- 9 oz. chicken fillet, chopped
- 1 teaspoon ground paprika
- 2 tablespoons sesame seeds
- ¼ teaspoon salt
- 1 cup chicken broth

Directions:

1. In the mixing bowl mix up chipotle chili, cilantro, chicken fillet, ground paprika, sesame seeds, and salt.
2. Then transfer the Ingredients in the instant pot and add chicken broth.

3. Cook the stew on manual mode (high pressure) for 10 minutes. Allow the natural pressure release for 10 minutes more.

Nutrition:

Calories 230

Fat 10.6

Fiber 2.6

Carbs 4.5

Protein 27.6

Keto Chili

Preparation Time: 10 minutes

Cooking Time: 25 minutes

Servings: 2 servings

Ingredients:

- ½ cup ground beef
- ½ teaspoon chili powder
- 1 teaspoon dried oregano
- ¼ cup crushed tomatoes
- 2 oz. scallions, diced
- 1 teaspoon avocado oil
- ¼ cup of water

Directions:

1. Mix up ground beef, chili powder, dried oregano, and scallions.
2. Then add avocado oil and stir the mixture.
3. Transfer it in the instant pot and cook on saute mode for 10 minutes.
4. Add water and crushed tomatoes. Stir the Ingredients with the help of the spatula until homogenous.
5. Close and seal the lid and cook the chili for 15 minutes on manual mode (high pressure).

Then make a quick pressure release.

Nutrition:

Calories 94

Fat 4.6

Fiber 2.4

Carbs 5.6

Protein 8

Pizza Soup

Preparation Time: 10 minutes

Cooking Time: 22 minutes

Servings: 3 servings

Ingredients:

- ¼ cup cremini mushrooms, sliced
- 1 teaspoon tomato paste
- 4 oz. Mozzarella, shredded
- ½ jalapeno pepper, sliced
- ½ teaspoon Italian seasoning
- 1 teaspoon coconut oil
- 5 oz. Italian sausages, chopped
- 1 cup of water

Directions:

1. Melt the coconut oil in the instant pot on saute mode.
2. Add mushrooms and cook them for 10 minutes.
3. After this, add chopped sausages, Italian seasoning, sliced jalapeno, and tomato paste.
4. Mix up the Ingredients well and add water.
5. Close and seal the lid and cook the soup on manual mode (high pressure) for 12 minutes.
6. Then make a quick pressure release and ladle the soup in the bowls. Top it with Mozzarella.

Nutrition:

Calories 289

Fat 23.2

Fiber 0.2

Carbs 2.5

Protein 17.7

Lamb Soup

Preparation Time: 10 minutes

Cooking Time: 25 minutes

Servings: 4 servings

Ingredients:

- ½ cup broccoli, roughly chopped
- 7 oz. lamb fillet, chopped
- ¼ teaspoon ground cumin
- ¼ daikon, chopped
- 2 bell peppers, chopped
- 1 tablespoon avocado oil
- 5 cups beef broth

Directions:

1. Saute the lamb fillet with avocado oil in the instant pot for 5 minutes.
2. Then add broccoli, ground cumin, and daikon, bell peppers, and beef broth.
3. Close and seal the lid.
4. Cook the soup on manual mode (high pressure) for 20 minutes.
5. Allow the natural pressure release.

Nutrition:

Calories 169

Fat 6

Fiber 1.3

Carbs 6.8

Protein 21

Minestrone Soup

Preparation Time: 10 minutes
Cooking Time: 25 minutes
Servings: 4 servings
Ingredients:

- 1 ½ cup ground pork
- ½ bell pepper, chopped
- 2 tablespoons chives, chopped
- 2 oz. celery stalk, chopped
- 1 teaspoon butter
- 1 teaspoon Italian seasonings
- 4 cups chicken broth
- ½ cup mushrooms, sliced

Directions:

1. Heat up butter on the saute mode for 2 minutes.
2. Add bell pepper. Cook the vegetable for 5 minutes.
3. Then stir them well and add mushrooms, celery stalk, and Italian seasonings. Stir well and cook for 5 minutes more.
4. Add ground pork, chives, and chicken broth.
5. Close and seal the lid.
6. Cook the soup on manual mode (high pressure) for 15 minutes. Make a quick pressure release.

Nutrition:

Calories 408

Fat 27.2

Fiber 0.6

Carbs 3

Protein 35.6

Chorizo Soup

Preparation Time: 10 minutes
Cooking Time: 17 minutes
Servings: 3 servings
Ingredients:

- 8 oz. chorizo, chopped
- 1 teaspoon tomato paste
- 4 oz. scallions, diced
- 1 tablespoon dried cilantro
- ½ teaspoon chili powder
- 1 teaspoon avocado oil
- 2 cups beef broth

Directions:

1. Heat up avocado oil on saute mode for 1 minute.
2. Add chorizo and cook it for 6 minutes, stir it from time to time.
3. Then add scallions, tomato paste, cilantro, and chili powder. Stir well.
4. Add beef broth.
5. Close and seal the lid.
6. Cook the soup on manual mode (high pressure) for 10 minutes. Make a quick pressure release.

Nutrition:

Calories 387

Fat 30.2

Fiber 1.3

Carbs 5.5

Protein 22.3

Red Feta Soup

Preparation Time: 10 minutes
Cooking Time: 25 minutes
Servings: 4 servings
Ingredients:

- 1 cup broccoli, chopped

- 1 teaspoon tomato paste
- ½ cup coconut cream
- 4 cups beef broth
- 1 teaspoon chili flakes
- 6 oz. feta, crumbled

Directions:

1. Put broccoli, tomato paste, coconut cream, and beef broth in the instant pot.
2. Add chili flakes and stir the mixture until it is red.
3. Then close and seal the lid and cook the soup for 8 minutes on manual mode (high pressure).
4. Then make a quick pressure release and open the lid.
5. Add feta cheese and saute the soup on saute mode for 5 minutes more.

Nutrition:

Calories 229

Fat 17.7

Fiber 1.3

Carbs 6.1

Protein 12.3

"Ramen" Soup

Preparation Time: 10 minutes

Cooking Time: 15 minutes

Servings: 2 servings

Ingredients:

- 1 zucchini, trimmed
- 2 cups chicken broth
- 2 eggs, boiled, peeled
- 1 tablespoon coconut aminos
- 5 oz. beef loin, strips
- 1 teaspoon chili flakes
- 1 tablespoon chives, chopped

- ½ teaspoon salt

Directions:

1. Put the beef loin strips in the instant pot.
2. Add chili flakes, salt, and chicken broth.
3. Close and seal the lid. Cook the **Ingredients:** on manual mode (high pressure) for 15 minutes. Make a quick pressure release and open the lid.
4. Then make the s from zucchini with the help of the spiralizer and add them in the soup.
5. Add chives and coconut aminos.
6. Then ladle the soup in the bowls and top with halved eggs.

Nutrition:

Calories 254

Fat 11.8

Fiber 1.1

Carbs 6.2

Protein 30.6

Beef Tagine

Preparation Time: 15 minutes

Cooking Time: 25 minutes

Servings: 6 servings

Ingredients:

- 1-pound beef fillet, chopped
- 1 eggplant, chopped
- 6 oz. scallions, chopped
- 1 teaspoon ground allspices
- 1 teaspoon Erythritol
- 1 teaspoon coconut oil
- 4 cups beef broth

Directions:

1. Put all Ingredients in the instant pot.

2. Close and seal the lid.
3. Cook the meal on manual mode (high pressure) for 25 minutes.
4. Then allow the natural pressure release for 15 minutes.

Nutrition:

Calories 146

Fat 5.3

Fiber 3.5

Carbs 8.8

Protein 16.7

Tomatillos Fish Stew

Preparation Time: 15 minutes

Cooking Time: 12 minutes

Servings: 2 servings

Ingredients:

- 2 tomatillos, chopped
- 10 oz. salmon fillet, chopped
- 1 teaspoon ground paprika
- ½ teaspoon ground turmeric
- 1 cup coconut cream
- ½ teaspoon salt

Directions:

1. Put all Ingredients in the instant pot.
2. Close and seal the lid.
3. Cook the fish stew on manual mode (high pressure) for 12 minutes.
4. Then allow the natural pressure release for 10 minutes.

Nutrition:

Calories 479

Fat 37.9

Fiber 3.8

Carbs 9.6

Protein 30.8

Chili Verde Soup

Preparation Time: 10 minutes

Cooking Time: 25 minutes

Servings: 4 servings

Ingredients:

- 2 oz. chili Verde sauce
- ½ cup Cheddar cheese, shredded
- 5 cups chicken broth
- 1-pound chicken breast, skinless, boneless
- 1 tablespoon dried cilantro

Directions:

1. Put chicken breast and chicken broth in the instant pot.
2. Add cilantro, close and seal the lid.
3. Then cook the Ingredients on manual (high pressure) for 15 minutes.
4. Make a quick pressure release and open the li.
5. Shred the chicken breast with the help of the fork.
6. Add dried cilantro and chili Verde sauce in the soup and cook it on saute mode for 10 minutes.
7. Then add dried cilantro and stir well.

Nutrition:

Calories 257

Fat 10.2

Fiber 0.2

Carbs 4

Protein 34.5

Pepper Stuffing Soup

Preparation Time: 10 minutes

Cooking Time: 14 minutes

Servings: 4 servings

Ingredients:

- 1 cup ground beef
- ½ cup cauliflower, shredded
- 1 teaspoon dried oregano
- ½ teaspoon salt
- 1 teaspoon tomato paste
- 1 teaspoon minced garlic
- 4 cups of water
- ¼ cup of coconut milk

Directions:

1. Put all Ingredients in the instant pot bowl and stir well.
2. Then close and seal the lid.
3. Cook the soup on manual mode (high pressure) for 14 minutes.
4. When the time of cooking is finished, make a quick pressure release and open the lid.

Nutrition:

Calories 106

Fat 7.7

Fiber 0.9

Carbs 2.2

Protein 7.3

Steak Soup

Preparation Time: 10 minutes

Cooking Time: 40 minutes

Servings: 5 servings

Ingredients:

- 5 oz. scallions, diced
- 1 tablespoon coconut oil
- 1 oz. daikon, diced
- 1-pound beef round steak, chopped
- 1 teaspoon dried thyme
- 5 cups of water
- ½ teaspoon ground black pepper

Directions:

1. Heat up coconut oil on saute mode for 2 minutes.
2. Add daikon and scallions.
3. After this, stir them well and add chopped beef steak, thyme, and ground black pepper.
4. Saute the Ingredients for 5 minutes more and then add water.
5. Close and seal the lid.
6. Cook the soup on manual mode (high pressure) for 35 minutes. Make a quick pressure release.

Nutrition:

Calories 232

Fat 11

Fiber 0.9

Carbs 2.5

Protein 29.5

Meat Spinach Stew

Preparation Time: 20 minutes

Cooking Time: 30 minutes

Servings: 4 servings

Ingredients:

- 2 cups spinach, chopped
- 1-pound beef sirloin, chopped
- 1 teaspoon allspices
- 3 cups chicken broth
- 1 cup of coconut milk
- 1 teaspoon coconut aminos

Directions:

1. Put all Ingredients in the instant pot.

2. Close and seal the lid.
3. After this, set the manual mode (high pressure) and cook the stew for 30 minutes.
4. When the cooking time is finished, allow the natural pressure release for 10 minutes.
5. Stir the stew gently before serving.

Nutrition:

Calories 383

Fat 22.2

Fiber 1.8

Carbs 5.1

Protein 39.9

Leek Soup

Preparation Time: 10 minutes

Cooking Time: 15 minutes

Servings: 4 servings

Ingredients:

- 7 oz. leek, chopped
- 2 oz. Monterey Jack cheese, shredded
- 1 teaspoon Italian seasonings
- ½ teaspoon salt
- 4 tablespoons butter
- 2 cups chicken broth

Directions:

1. Heat up butter in the instant pot for 4 minutes.
2. Then add chopped leek, salt, and Italian seasonings.
3. Cook the leek on saute mode for 5 minutes. Stir the vegetables from time to time.
4. After this, add chicken broth and close the lid.
5. Cook the soup on saute mode for 10 minutes.

6. Then add shredded cheese and stir it till the cheese is melted.
7. The soup is cooked.

Nutrition:

Calories 208

Fat 17

Fiber 0.9

Carbs 7.7

Protein 6.8

Asparagus Soup

Preparation Time: 10 minutes

Cooking Time: 17 minutes

Servings: 4 servings

Ingredients:

- 1 cup asparagus, chopped
- 2 cups of coconut milk
- 1 teaspoon salt
- ½ teaspoon cayenne pepper
- 3 oz. scallions, diced
- 1 teaspoon olive oil

Directions:

1. Saute the chopped asparagus, scallions, and olive oil in the instant pot for 7 minutes.
2. Then stir the vegetables well and add cayenne pepper, salt, and coconut milk
3. Cook the soup on manual mode (high pressure) for 10 minutes.
4. After this, make a quick pressure release and open the lid.
5. Blend the soup until you get the creamy texture.

Nutrition:

Calories 300 Fat 29.9

Fiber 4 Carbs 9.6 Protein 3.9

Bok Choy Soup

Preparation Time: 5 minutes

Cooking Time: 2 minutes

Servings: 1 serving

Ingredients:

- 1 bok choy stalk, chopped
- ¼ teaspoon nutritional yeast
- ½ teaspoon onion powder
- ¼ teaspoon chili flakes
- 1 cup chicken broth

Directions:

1. Put all Ingredients from the list above in the instant pot.
2. Close and seal the lid and cook the soup on manual (high pressure) for 2 minutes.
3. Make a quick pressure release.

Nutrition:

Calories 58

Fat 1.7

Fiber 1.3

Carbs 4.5

Protein 6.9

Curry Kale Soup

Preparation Time: 10 minutes

Cooking Time: 15 minutes

Servings: 3 servings

Ingredients:

- 2 cups kale
- 1 tablespoon fresh cilantro
- 1 teaspoon curry paste
- ½ cup heavy cream
- ½ cup ground chicken
- 1 teaspoon almond butter
- ½ teaspoon salt 1 cup chicken stock

Directions:

1. Blend the kale until smooth and put it in the instant pot.
2. Add cilantro, almond butter, and ground chicken. Saute the mixture for 5 minutes.
3. Meanwhile, in the shallow bowl, mix up curry paste and heavy cream. When the liquid is smooth, pour it in the instant pot.
4. Add chicken stock and salt, and close the lid.
5. Cook the soup on manual (high pressure) for 10 minutes. Make a quick pressure release.

Nutrition:

Calories 183

Fat 13.3

Fiber 1.2

Carbs 7

Protein 9.9

Turmeric Rutabaga Soup

Preparation Time: 15 minutes

Cooking Time: 15 minutes

Servings: 5 servings

Ingredients:

- 3 turnips, chopped
- 1 teaspoon ginger paste
- 2 oz. celery, chopped
- 1 teaspoon ground turmeric
- 1 teaspoon minced garlic
- 2 cups of coconut milk
- 1 cup beef broth
- 2 oz. bell pepper, chopped

Directions:

1. Place all Ingredients in the instant pot and stir them gently.

2. Then close and seal the lid; set manual mode (high pressure) and cook the soup for 15 minutes.
3. Then allow the natural pressure release for 10 minutes and ladle the soup into the serving bowls.

Nutrition:

Calories 255

Fat 23.2

Fiber 3.6

Carbs 11.4

Protein 4

Cream of Mushrooms Soup

Preparation Time: 10 minutes

Cooking Time: 35 minutes

Servings: 6 servings

Ingredients:

- 3 cups cremini mushrooms, sliced
- 1 cup of coconut milk
- 1 tablespoon almond flour
- 1 teaspoon salt
- 1 teaspoon ground black pepper
- 4 cups chicken broth
- 3 tablespoons butter

Directions:

1. Melt the butter on saute mode.
2. Add cremini mushrooms and saute them for 10 minutes. Stir them with the help of the spatula from time to time.
3. After this, in the bowl mix up salt, almond flour, and ground black pepper. Add coconut milk and stir the liquid.
4. Pour the liquid over the mushrooms.

5. Add chicken broth. Close and seal the lid.
6. Cook the soup on saute mode for 25 minutes.

Nutrition:

Calories 206

Fat 18.6

Fiber 1.7

Carbs 5.5

Protein 6.2

Flu Soup

Preparation Time: 10 minutes

Cooking Time: 15 minutes

Servings: 4 servings

Ingredients:

- 1 cup mushrooms, chopped
- 1 cup spinach, chopped
- 3 oz. scallions, diced
- 2 oz. Cheddar cheese, shredded
- 1 teaspoon cayenne pepper
- 1 cup organic almond milk
- 2 cups chicken broth
- ½ teaspoon salt

Directions:

1. Put all Ingredients in the instant pot and close the lid.
2. Set the manual mode (high pressure) and cook the soup for 15 minutes.
3. Make a quick pressure release.
4. Blend the soup with the help of the immersion blender.
5. When the soup will get smooth texture – it is cooked.

Nutrition:

Calories 228 Fat 19.9 Fiber 2.3

Carbs 6.6 Protein 8.5

Jalapeno Soup

Preparation Time: 10 minutes
Cooking Time: 10 minutes
Servings: 4 servings
Ingredients:

- 2 jalapeno peppers, sliced
- 3 oz. pancetta, chopped
- ½ cup heavy cream
- 2 cups of water
- ½ cup Monterey jack cheese, shredded
- ½ teaspoon garlic powder
- 1 teaspoon coconut oil
- ½ teaspoon smoked paprika

Directions:

1. Toss pancetta in the instant pot, add coconut oil and cook it for 4 minutes on saute mode. Stir it from time to time.
2. After this, add sliced jalapenos, garlic powder, and smoked paprika.
3. Stir the Ingredients for 1 minute.
4. Add heavy cream and water.
5. Then add Monterey Jack cheese and stir the soup well.
6. Close and seal the lid; cook the soup for 5 minutes on manual mode (high pressure); make a quick pressure release.

Nutrition:

Calories 234

Fat 20

Fiber 0.4

Carbs 1.7

Protein 11.8

Garden Soup

Preparation Time: 20 minutes
Cooking Time: 29 minutes
Servings: 5 servings
Ingredients:

- ½ cup cauliflower florets
- 1 cup kale, chopped
- 1 garlic clove, diced
- 1 tablespoon olive oil
- 1 teaspoon sea salt
- 6 cups beef broth
- 2 tablespoons chives, chopped

Directions:

1. Heat up olive oil in the instant pot on saute mode for 2 minutes and add clove.
2. Cook the vegetables for 2 minutes and stir well.
3. Add kale, cauliflower, and sea salt, chives, and beef broth.
4. Close and seal the lid.
5. Cook the soup on manual mode (high pressure) for 5 minutes.
6. Then make a quick pressure release and open the lid.
7. Ladle the soup into the bowls.

Nutrition:

Calories 80 Fat 4.5

Fiber 0.5 Carbs 2.3 Protein 6.5

Shirataki Noodle Soup

Preparation Time: 25 minutes
Cooking Time: 15 minutes
Servings: 2 servings
Ingredients:

- 2 oz. shirataki noodles
- 2 cups of water
- 6 oz. chicken fillet, chopped

- 1 teaspoon salt
- 1 tablespoon coconut aminos

Directions:
1. Pour water in the instant pot bowl.
2. Add salt and chopped chicken fillet. Close and seal the lid.
3. Cook the Ingredients on manual mode (high pressure) for 15 minutes. Allow the natural pressure release for 10 minutes.
4. After this, add shirataki noodles and coconut aminos.
5. Leave the soup for 10 minutes to rest.

Nutrition:
Calories 175
Fat 6.3
Fiber 3
Carbs 1.5
Protein 24.8

Cordon Blue Soup
Preparation Time: 15 minutes
Cooking Time: 6 minutes
Servings: 4 servings
Ingredients:

- 4 cups chicken broth
- 7 oz. ham, chopped
- 3 oz. Mozzarella cheese, shredded
- 1 teaspoon ground black pepper
- ½ teaspoon salt
- 2 tablespoons ricotta cheese
- 2 oz. scallions, chopped

Directions:
1. Put all Ingredients in the instant pot bowl and stir gently.

2. Close and seal the lid; cook the soup on manual mode (high pressure) for 6 minutes.
3. Then allow the natural pressure release for 10 minutes and ladle the soup into the bowls.

Nutrition:
Calories 196
Fat 10.1
Fiber 1.2
Carbs 5.3
Protein 20.3

Bacon Soup
Preparation Time: 10 minutes
Cooking Time: 20 minutes
Servings: 4 servings
Ingredients:

- 3 oz. bacon, chopped
- 1 cup cheddar cheese, shredded
- 1 tablespoon scallions, chopped
- 3 cups beef broth 1 cup of coconut milk
- 1 teaspoon curry powder

Directions:
1. Heat up the instant pot on saute mode for 3 minutes and add bacon.
2. Cook it for 5 minutes. Stir it from time to time.
3. Then add scallions and curry powder. Cook the Ingredients for 5 minutes more. Stir them from time to time.
4. After this, add coconut milk and beef broth.
5. Add cheddar cheese and stir the soup well.

6. Cook it on manual mode (high pressure) for 10 minutes. Make a quick pressure release.
7. Mix up the soup well before serving.

Nutrition:

calories 398 fat 33.6 fiber 1.5 carbs 5.1 protein 20

Paprika Zucchini Soup

Preparation Time: 10 minutes

Cooking Time: 1 minute

Servings: 2 servings

Ingredients:

- 1 zucchini, grated
- 1 teaspoon ground paprika
- ½ teaspoon cayenne pepper
- ½ cup of coconut milk
- 1 cup beef broth
- 1 tablespoon dried cilantro
- 1 oz. Parmesan, grated

Directions:

1. Put the grated zucchini, paprika, cayenne pepper, coconut milk, beef broth, and dried cilantro in the instant pot.
2. Close and seal the lid.
3. Cook the soup on manual (high pressure) for 1 minute. Make a quick pressure release.
4. Ladle the soup in the serving bowls and top with parmesan.

Nutrition:

calories 223

fat 18.4

fiber 2.9

carbs 8.4

protein 9.7

Egg Drop Soup

Preparation Time: 5 minutes

Cooking Time: 10 minutes

Servings: 4 servings

Ingredients:

- 4 cups chicken broth
- 2 tablespoons fresh dill, chopped
- 2 eggs, beaten
- 1 teaspoon salt

Directions:

1. Pour chicken broth in the instant pot.
2. Add salt and bring it to boil on Saute mode.
3. Then add beaten eggs and stir the liquid well.
4. Add dill and saute it for 5 minutes.
5. The soup is cooked.

Nutrition:

calories 74

fat 3.6

fiber 0.2

carbs 2

protein 7.9

Buffalo Style Soup

Preparation Time: 7 minutes

Cooking Time: 10 minutes

Servings: 2 servings

Ingredients:

- 6 oz. chicken, cooked
- 2 oz. Mozzarella, shredded
- 4 tablespoons coconut milk
- ¼ teaspoon white pepper
- ¾ teaspoon salt
- 2 tablespoons keto Buffalo sauce
- 1 oz. celery stalk, chopped
- 1 cup of water

Directions:

1. Place the chopped celery stalk, water, salt, white pepper, coconut milk, and Mozzarella in the instant pot. Stir it gently.
2. Set the "Manual" mode (High pressure) and turn on the timer for 7 minutes.
3. Shred the cooked chicken and combine it together with Buffalo Sauce.
4. Make quick pressure release and transfer the soup on the bowls.
5. Add shredded chicken and stir it.

Nutrition:

calories 287

fat 14.8

fiber 1.5

carbs 4.3

protein 33.5

CHAPTER 5:

Poultry

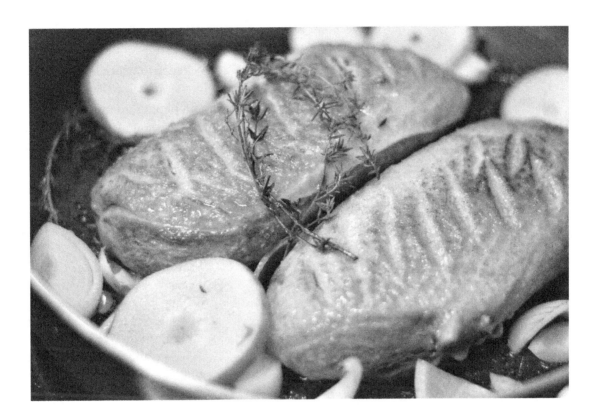

Country-Style Chicken Stew

Preparation Time: 20 minutes
Cooking Time: 1 hour
Servings: 6
Ingredients:

- 1 pound chicken thighs
- 2 tablespoons butter, room temperature
- 1/2 pound carrots, chopped
- 1 bell pepper, chopped
- 1 chile pepper, deveined and minced
- 1 cup tomato puree
- Kosher salt and ground black pepper, to taste
- 1/2 teaspoon smoked paprika
- 1 onion, finely chopped
- 1 teaspoon garlic, sliced
- 4 cups vegetable broth
- 1 teaspoon dried basil
- 1 celery, chopped

Directions:

1. Melt the butter in a stockpot over medium-high flame. Sweat the onion and garlic until just tender and fragrant.
2. Reduce the heat to medium-low. Stir in the broth, chicken thighs, and basil; bring to a rolling boil.
3. Add in the remaining Ingredients. Partially cover and let it simmer for 45 to 50 minutes. Shred the meat, discarding the bones; add the chicken back to the pot.

Nutrition:
280 Calories 14.7g Fat
2.5g Carbs 25.6g Protein
2.5g Fiber

Autumn Chicken Soup with Root Vegetables

Preparation Time: 10 minutes
Cooking Time: 25 minutes
Servings: 4
Ingredients: 4 cups chicken broth

- 1 cup full-fat milk
- 1 cup double cream
- 1/2 cup turnip, chopped
- 2 chicken drumsticks, boneless and cut into small pieces
- Salt and pepper, to taste
- 1 tablespoon butter
- 1 teaspoon garlic, finely minced
- 1 carrot, chopped
- 1/2 parsnip, chopped
- 1/2 celery - 1 whole egg

Directions:

1. Melt the butter in a heavy-bottomed pot over medium-high heat; sauté the garlic until aromatic or about 1 minute. Add in the vegetables and continue to cook until they've softened.
2. Add in the chicken and cook until it is no longer pink for about 4 minutes. Season with salt and pepper.
3. Pour in the chicken broth, milk, and heavy cream and bring it to a boil.
4. Reduce the heat to. Partially cover and continue to simmer for 20 to 25 minutes longer. Afterwards, fold the beaten egg and stir until it is well incorporated.

Nutrition: 342 Calories 22.4g Fat
6.3g Carbs 25.2g Protein 1.3g Fiber

Panna Cotta with Chicken and Bleu d' Auvergne

Preparation Time: 10 minutes

Cooking Time: 20 minutes

Servings:

Ingredients:

- 2 chicken legs, boneless and skinless
- 1 tablespoon avocado oil
- 2 teaspoons granular erythritol
- 3 tablespoons water
- 1 cup Bleu d' Auvergne, crumbled
- 2 gelatin sheets
- 3/4 cup double cream
- Salt and cayenne pepper, to your liking

Directions:

1. Heat the oil in a frying pan over medium-high heat; fry the chicken for about 10 minutes.
2. Soak the gelatin sheets in cold water. Cook with the cream, erythritol, water, and Bleu d' Auvergne.
3. Season with salt and pepper and let it simmer over the low heat, stirring for about 3 minutes. Spoon the mixture into four ramekins.

Nutrition:

306 Calories

18.3g Fat

4.7g Carbs

29.5g Protein

0g Fiber

Breaded Chicken Fillets

Preparation Time: 15 minutes

Cooking Time: 30 minutes

Servings: 4

Ingredients:

- 1 pound chicken fillets
- 3 bell peppers, quartered lengthwise
- 1/3 cup Romano cheese
- 2 teaspoons olive oil
- 1 garlic clove, minced
- Kosher salt and ground black pepper, to taste
- 1/3 cup crushed pork rinds

Directions:

1. Start by preheating your oven to 410 degrees F.
2. Mix the crushed pork rinds, Romano cheese, olive oil and minced garlic. Dredge the chicken into this mixture.
3. Place the chicken in a lightly greased baking dish. Season with salt and black pepper to taste.
4. Scatter the peppers around the chicken and bake in the preheated oven for 20 to 25 minutes or until thoroughly cooked.

Nutrition:

367 Calories

16.9g Fat

6g Carbs

43g Protein

0.7g Fiber

Chicken Drumsticks with Broccoli and Cheese

Preparation Time: 40 minutes

Cooking Time: 1 hour 15 minutes

Servings: 4

Ingredients:

- 1 pound chicken drumsticks
- 1 pound broccoli, broken into florets
- 2 cups cheddar cheese, shredded
- 1/2 teaspoon dried oregano
- 1/2 teaspoon dried basil
- 3 tablespoons olive oil
- 1 celery, sliced
- 1 cup green onions, chopped
- 1 teaspoon minced green garlic

Directions:

1. Roast the chicken drumsticks in the preheated oven at 380 degrees F for 30 to 35 minutes. Add in the broccoli, celery, green onions, and green garlic.
2. Add in the oregano, basil and olive oil; roast an additional 15 minutes.

Nutrition:

533 Calories

40.2g Fat

5.4g Carbs

35.1g Protein

3.5g Fiber

Turkey Ham and Mozzarella Pate

Preparation Time: 5 minutes

Cooking Time: 10 minutes

Servings: 6

Ingredients:

- 4 ounces turkey ham, chopped
- 2 tablespoons fresh parsley, roughly chopped
- 2 tablespoons flaxseed meal
- 4 ounces mozzarella cheese, crumbled
- 2 tablespoons sunflower seeds

Directions:

1. Thoroughly combine the Ingredients, except for the sunflower seeds, in your food processor.
2. Spoon the mixture into a serving bowl and scatter the sunflower seeds over the top.

Nutrition:

212 Calories

18.8g Fat

2g Carbs

10.6g Protein

1.6g Fiber

Greek-Style Saucy Chicken Drumettes

Preparation Time: 25 minutes

Cooking Time: 50 minutes

Servings: 6

Ingredients:

- 1 ½ pounds chicken drumettes
- 1/2 cup port wine
- 1/2 cup onions, chopped
- 2 garlic cloves, minced
- 1 teaspoon tzatziki spice mix
- 1 cup double cream
- 2 tablespoons butter
- Sea salt and crushed mixed peppercorns, to season

Directions:

1. Melt the butter in an oven-proof skillet over a moderate heat; then, cook the chicken for about 8 minutes.
2. Add in the onions, garlic, wine, tzatziki spice mix, double cream, salt, and pepper.
3. Bake in the preheated oven at 390 degrees F for 35 to 40 minutes (a meat thermometer should register 165 degrees F).

Nutrition:

333 Calories

20.2g Fat

2g Carbs

33.5g Protein

0.2g Fiber

Chicken with Avocado Sauce

Preparation Time: 10 minutes

Cooking Time: 20 minutes

Servings: 4

Ingredients:

- 8 chicken wings, boneless, cut into bite-size chunks
- 2 tablespoons olive oil
- Sea salt and pepper, to your liking
- 2 eggs
- 1 teaspoon onion powder
- 1 teaspoon hot paprika
- 1/3 teaspoon mustard seeds
- 1/3 cup almond meal

For the Sauce:

- 1/2 cup mayonnaise
- 1/2 medium avocado
- 1/2 teaspoon sea salt
- 1 teaspoon green garlic, minced

Directions:

1. Pat dry the chicken wings with a paper towel.
2. Thoroughly combine the almond meal, salt, pepper, onion powder, paprika, and mustard seeds.
3. Whisk the eggs in a separate dish. Dredge the chicken chunks into the whisked eggs, then in the almond meal mixture.
4. In a frying pan, heat the oil over a moderate heat; once hot, fry the chicken for about 10 minutes, stirring continuously to ensure even cooking.
5. Make the sauce by whisking all of the sauce Ingredients.

Nutrition:

370 Calories

25g Fat

4.1g Carbs

31.4g Protein

2.6g Fiber

Old-Fashioned Turkey Chowder

Preparation Time: 15 minutes

Cooking Time: 35 minutes

Servings: 4

Ingredients:

- 2 tablespoons olive oil
- 2 tablespoons yellow onions, chopped
- 2 cloves garlic, roughly chopped
- 1/2 pound leftover roast turkey, shredded and skin removed
- 1 teaspoon Mediterranean spice mix
- 3 cups chicken bone broth
- 1 ½ cups milk
- 1/2 cup double cream

- 1 egg, lightly beaten
- 2 tablespoons dry sherry

Directions:

1. Heat the olive oil in a heavy-bottomed pot over a moderate flame. Sauté the onion and garlic until they've softened.
2. Stir in the leftover roast turkey, Mediterranean spice mix, and chicken bone broth; bring to a rapid boil. Partially cover and continue to cook for 20 to 25 minutes.
3. Turn the heat to simmer. Pour in the milk and double cream and continue to cook until it has reduced slightly.
4. Fold in the egg and dry sherry; continue to simmer, stirring frequently, for a further 2 minutes.

Nutrition:

350 Calories

25.8g Fat

5.5g Carbs

20g Protein

0.1g Fiber

Duck and Eggplant Casserole

Preparation Time: 10 minutes

Cooking Time: 45 minutes

Servings: 4

Ingredients:

- 1 pound ground duck meat
- 1 ½ tablespoons ghee, melted
- 1/3 cup double cream
- 1/2 pound eggplant, peeled and sliced
- 1 ½ cups almond flour

- Salt and black pepper, to taste
- 1/2 teaspoon fennel seeds
- 1/2 teaspoon oregano, dried
- 8 eggs

Directions:

1. Mix the almond flour with salt, black, fennel seeds, and oregano. Fold in one egg and the melted ghee and whisk to combine well.
2. Press the crust into the bottom of a lightly-oiled pie pan. Cook the ground duck until no longer pink for about 3 minutes, stirring continuously.
3. Whisk the remaining eggs and double cream. Fold in the browned meat and stir until everything is well incorporated. Pour the mixture into the prepared crust. Top with the eggplant slices.
4. Bake for about 40 minutes. Cut into four pieces.

Nutrition:

562 Calories

49.5g Fat

6.7g Carbs

22.5g Protein

2.1g Fiber

Herbed Chicken Breasts

Preparation Time: 10 minutes

Cooking Time: 40 minutes

Servings: 8

Ingredients:

- 4 chicken breasts, skinless and boneless
- 1 Italian pepper, deveined and thinly sliced

- 10 black olives, pitted
- 1 ½ cups vegetable broth
- 2 garlic cloves, pressed
- 2 tablespoons olive oil
- 1 tablespoon Old Sub Sailor
- Salt, to taste

Directions:

1. Rub the chicken with the garlic and Old Sub Sailor; salt to taste. Heat the oil in a frying pan over a moderately high heat.
2. Sear the chicken until it is browned on all sides, about 5 minutes.
3. Add in the pepper, olives, and vegetable broth and bring it to boil. Reduce the heat simmer and continue to cook, partially covered, for 30 to 35 minutes.

Nutrition:

306 Calories

17.8g Fat

3.1g Carbs

31.7g Protein

0.2g Fiber

Cheese and Prosciutto Chicken Roulade

Preparation Time: 15 minutes

Cooking Time: 35 minutes

Servings: 2

Ingredients:

- 1/2 cup Ricotta cheese
- 4 slices of prosciutto
- 1 pound chicken fillet
- 1 tablespoon fresh coriander, chopped

- Salt and ground black pepper, to taste pepper
- 1 teaspoon cayenne pepper

Directions:

1. Season the chicken fillet with salt and pepper. Spread the Ricotta cheese over the chicken fillet; sprinkle with the fresh coriander.
2. Roll up and cut into 4 pieces. Wrap each piece with one slice of prosciutto; secure with a kitchen twine.
3. Place the wrapped chicken in a parchment-lined baking pan. Now, bake in the preheated oven at 385 degrees F for about 30 minutes.

Nutrition:

499 Calories

18.9g Fat

5.7g Carbs

41.6g Protein

0.6g Fiber

Boozy Glazed Chicken

Preparation Time: 40 minutes

Cooking Time: 1 hour + marinating time

Servings: 4

Ingredients:

- 2 pounds chicken drumettes
- 2 tablespoons ghee, at room temperature
- Sea salt and ground black pepper, to taste
- 1 teaspoon Mediterranean seasoning mix
- 2 vine-ripened tomatoes, pureed
- 3/4 cup rum

- 3 tablespoons coconut aminos
- A few drops of liquid Stevia
- 1 teaspoon chile peppers, minced
- 1 tablespoon minced fresh ginger
- 1 teaspoon ground cardamom
- 2 tablespoons fresh lemon juice, plus wedges for serving

Directions:

1. Toss the chicken with the melted ghee, salt, black pepper, and Mediterranean seasoning mix until well coated on all sides.
2. In another bowl, thoroughly combine the pureed tomato puree, rum, coconut aminos, Stevia, chile peppers, ginger, cardamom, and lemon juice.
3. Pour the tomato mixture over the chicken drumettes; let it marinate for 2 hours. Bake in the preheated oven at 410 degrees F for about 45 minutes.
4. Add in the reserved marinade and place under the preheated broiler for 10 minutes.

Nutrition:
307 Calories 12.1g Fat
2.7g Carbs
33.6g Protein
1.5g Fiber

Festive Turkey Rouladen
Preparation Time: 15 minutes
Cooking Time: 30 minutes
Servings: 5
Ingredients:

- 2 pounds turkey fillet, marinated and cut into 10 pieces

- 10 strips prosciutto
- 1/2 teaspoon chili powder
- 1 teaspoon marjoram
- 1 sprig rosemary, finely chopped
- 2 tablespoons dry white wine
- 1 teaspoon garlic, finely minced
- 1 ½ tablespoons butter, room temperature
- 1 tablespoon Dijon mustard
- Sea salt and freshly ground black pepper, to your liking

Directions:

1. Start by preheating your oven to 430 degrees F.
2. Pat the turkey dry and cook in hot butter for about 3 minutes per side. Add in the mustard, chili powder, marjoram, rosemary, wine, and garlic.
3. Continue to cook for 2 minutes more. Wrap each turkey piece into one prosciutto strip and secure with toothpicks.
4. Roast in the preheated oven for about 30 minutes.

Nutrition:
286 Calories
9.7g Fat
6.9g Carbs
39.9g Protein
0.3g Fiber

Pan-Fried Chorizo Sausage
Preparation Time: 10 minutes
Cooking Time: 20 minutes
Servings: 4
Ingredients:

- 16 ounces smoked turkey chorizo

- 1 ½ cups Asiago cheese, grated
- 1 teaspoon oregano
- 1 teaspoon basil
- 1 cup tomato puree
- 4 scallion stalks, chopped
- 1 teaspoon garlic paste
- Sea salt and ground black pepper, to taste
- 1 tablespoon dry sherry
- 1 tablespoon extra-virgin olive oil
- 2 tablespoons fresh coriander, roughly chopped

Directions:

1. Heat the oil in a frying pan over moderately high heat. Now, brown the turkey chorizo, crumbling with a fork for about 5 minutes.
2. Add in the other Ingredients, except for cheese; continue to cook for 10 minutes more or until cooked through.

Nutrition:

330 Calories

17.2g Fat

4.5g Carbs

34.4g Protein

1.6g Fiber

Chinese Bok Choy and Turkey Soup

Preparation Time: 15 minutes

Cooking Time: 40 minutes

Servings: 8

Ingredients:

- 1/2 pound baby Bok choy, sliced into quarters lengthwise
- 2 pounds turkey carcass

- 1 tablespoon olive oil
- 1/2 cup leeks, chopped
- 1 celery rib, chopped
- 2 carrots, sliced
- 6 cups turkey stock
- Himalayan salt and black pepper, to taste

Directions:

1. In a heavy-bottomed pot, heat the olive oil until sizzling. Once hot, sauté the celery, carrots, leek and Bok choy for about 6 minutes.
2. Add the salt, pepper, turkey, and stock; bring to a boil.
3. Turn the heat to simmer. Continue to cook, partially covered, for about 35 minutes.

Nutrition:

211 Calories 11.8g Fat

3.1g Carbs

23.7g Protein

0.9g Fiber

Herby Chicken Meatloaf

Preparation Time: 20 minutes

Cooking Time: 30 minutes

Servings: 6

Ingredients:

- 2 ½ lb. ground chicken
- 3 tbsp flaxseed meal
- 2 large eggs
- 2 tbsp olive oil
- 1 lemon,1 tbsp juiced
- ¼ cup chopped parsley
- ¼ cup chopped oregano
- 4 garlic cloves, minced
- Lemon slices to garnish

Directions:

1. Preheat oven to 400 F. In a bowl, combine ground chicken and flaxseed meal; set aside. In a small bowl, whisk the eggs with olive oil, lemon juice, parsley, oregano, and garlic.
2. Pour the mixture onto the chicken mixture and mix well. Spoon into a greased loaf pan and press to fit. Bake for 40 minutes.
3. Remove the pan, drain the liquid, and let cool a bit. Slice, garnish with lemon slices, and serve.

Nutrition:
Cal 362
Net Carbs 1.3g
Fat 24g
Protein 35g

Lovely Pulled Chicken Egg Bites
Preparation Time: 15 minutes
Cooking Time: 30 minutes
Servings: 4
Ingredients:

- 2 tbsp butter
- 1 chicken breast
- 2 tbsp chopped green onions
- ½ tsp red chili flakes
- 12 eggs
- ¼ cup grated Monterey Jack

Directions:

1. Preheat oven to 400 F. Line a 12-hole muffin tin with cupcake liners. Melt butter in a skillet over medium heat and cook the chicken until brown on each side, 10 minutes.

2. Transfer to a plate and shred with 2 forks. Divide between muffin holes along with green onions and red chili flakes.
3. Crack an egg into each muffin hole and scatter the cheese on top. Bake for 15 minutes until eggs set. Serve.

Nutrition:
Cal 393
Net Carbs 0.5g
Fat 27g
Protein 34g

Creamy Mustard Chicken with Shirataki
Preparation Time: 20 minutes
Cooking Time: 30 minutes
Servings: 4
Ingredients:

- 2 (8 oz.) packs angel hair shirataki
- 4 chicken breasts, cut into strips
- 1 cup chopped mustard greens
- 1 yellow bell pepper, sliced
- 1 tbsp olive oil
- 1 yellow onion, finely sliced
- 1 garlic clove, minced
- 1 tbsp wholegrain mustard
- 5 tbsp heavy cream
- 1 tbsp chopped parsley

Directions:

1. Boil 2 cups of water in a medium pot.
2. Strain the shirataki pasta and rinse well under hot running water. Allow proper draining and pour the shirataki pasta into the boiling water.

3. Cook for 3 minutes and strain again. Place a dry skillet and stir-fry the shirataki pasta until visibly dry, 1-2 minutes; set aside.

4. Heat olive oil in a skillet, season the chicken with salt and pepper and cook for 8-10 minutes; set aside. Stir in onion, bell pepper, and garlic and cook until softened, 5 minutes.

5. Mix in mustard and heavy cream; simmer for 2 minutes and mix in the chicken and mustard greens for 2 minutes. Stir in shirataki pasta, garnish with parsley and serve.

Nutrition:

Cal 692

Net Carbs 15g

Fats 38g

Protein 65g

CHAPTER 6:

Beef Recipes

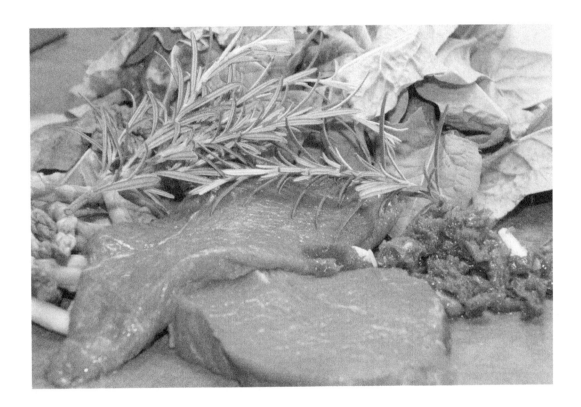

Mustard-Lemon Beef

Preparation Time: 15 minutes

Cooking Time: 25 minutes

Servings: 4

Ingredients:

- 2 tbsp olive oil
- 1 tbsp fresh rosemary, chopped
- 2 garlic cloves, minced
- 1 ½ lb. beef rump steak, thinly sliced
- Salt and black pepper to taste
- 1 shallot, chopped
- ½ cup heavy cream
- ½ cup beef stock
- 1 tbsp mustard
- 2 tsp Worcestershire sauce
- 2 tsp lemon juice
- 1 tsp erythritol
- 2 tbsp butter
- 1 tbsp fresh rosemary, chopped
- 1 tbsp fresh thyme, chopped

Directions:

1. In a bowl, combine 1 tbsp of oil with black pepper, garlic, rosemary, and salt. Toss in the beef to coat and set aside for some minutes. Heat a pan with the rest of the oil over medium heat, place in the beef steak, and cook for 6 minutes, flipping halfway through. Set aside and keep warm.
2. Melt the butter in the pan. Add in the shallot and cook for 3 minutes. Stir in the stock, Worcestershire sauce, erythritol, thyme, cream, mustard, and rosemary and cook for 8 minutes. Mix in the lemon juice, pepper, and salt. Arrange the beef slices on serving plates, sprinkle over the sauce, and enjoy!

Nutrition: Kcal 435 Fat 30g
Net Carbs 5g Protein 32g

Ribeye Steak with Shitake Mushrooms

Preparation Time: 10 minutes

Cooking Time: 25 minutes

Servings: 4

Ingredients:

- 1 lb. ribeye steaks
- 1 tbsp butter
- 2 tbsp olive oil
- 1 cup shitake mushrooms, sliced
- Salt and black pepper to taste
- 2 tbsp fresh parsley, chopped

Directions:

1. Heat the olive oil in a pan over medium heat. Rub the steaks with salt and black pepper and cook about 4 minutes per side; reserve.
2. Melt the butter in the pan and cook the shitakes for 4 minutes. Scatter the parsley over and pour the mixture over the steaks to serve.

Nutrition:

Calories: 406 Fat: 21g

Carb: 11g, Protein: 10g

Parsley Beef Burgers

Preparation Time: 10 minutes

Cooking Time: 25 minutes

Servings: 6

Ingredients:

- 2 lb. ground beef
- 1 tbsp onion flakes
- ¾ cup almond flour

- ¼ cup beef broth
- 2 tbsp fresh parsley, chopped
- 1 tbsp Worcestershire sauce

Directions:

1. Combine all ingredients in a bowl. Mix well with your hands and make 6 patties out of the mixture. Arrange on a lined baking sheet. Bake at 370°F for about 18 minutes, until nice and crispy. Serve.

Nutrition:

Kcal 354

Fat: 28g

Net Carbs: 2.5g

Protein: 27g

Beef Cauliflower Curry

Preparation Time: 15 minutes

Cooking Time: 26 minutes

Servings: 6

Ingredients:

- 1 tbsp olive oil
- 1 ½ lb. ground beef
- 1 tbsp ginger paste
- 1 tsp garam masala
- 1 (7 oz.) can whole tomatoes
- 1 head cauliflower, cut into florets
- Salt to taste
- 2 garlic cloves, minced
- ½ tsp hot paprika

Directions:

2. Heat oil in a saucepan over medium heat. Add the beef, ginger, garlic, garam masala, paprika, and salt and cook for 5 minutes while breaking any lumps. Stir in the tomatoes and cauliflower. Cook covered for 6 minutes.

3. Add ½ cup water and bring to a boil. Simmer for 10 minutes or until the water has reduced by half. Spoon the curry into serving bowls and serve with shirataki rice.

Nutrition:

Kcal 374

Fat 33g

Net Carbs 2g

Protein 22g

Italian Beef Ragout

Preparation Time: 40 minutes

Cooking Time: 1 hour 55 minutes

Servings: 4

Ingredients:

- 1 lb. chuck steak, cubed
- 2 tbsp olive oil
- Salt and black pepper to taste
- 2 tbsp almond flour
- 1 onion, diced
- ½ cup dry white wine
- 1 red bell pepper, seeded and diced
- 2 tsp Worcestershire sauce
- 4 oz. tomato puree
- 3 tsp smoked paprika
- 1 cup beef broth
- 2 tbsp fresh thyme, chopped

Directions:

1. Lightly dredge the meat in the almond flour. Place a large skillet over medium heat, add the olive oil to heat and then sauté the onion and bell pepper for 3 minutes. Stir in paprika.

2. Add the beef and cook for 10 minutes in total while turning them halfway. Stir in white wine and let it reduce by half, about 3 minutes.

3. Add in Worcestershire sauce, tomato puree, beef broth, salt, and pepper. Let the mixture boil for 2 minutes, reduce the heat, and let simmer for 1 ½ hours, stirring often. Serve garnished with thyme.

Nutrition:

Calories: 129.2

Fat: 4.7g

Carb: 16.3g,

Protein: 27g

Beef Meatballs

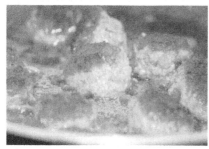

Preparation Time: 23 minutes

Cooking Time: 35 minutes

Servings: 4

Ingredients:

- ½ cup pork rinds, crushed
- 1 egg
- Salt and black pepper to taste
- 1 ½ lb. ground beef
- 10 oz. canned onion soup
- 1 tbsp almond flour
- ¼ cup free-sugar ketchup
- 3 tsp Worcestershire sauce
- ½ tsp dry mustard

Directions:

1. In a bowl, combine 1/3 cup of the onion soup with the beef, pepper, pork rinds, egg, and salt. Shape the

mixture into 12 meatballs. Heat a greased pan over medium heat. Brown the meatballs for 12 minutes.

2. In a separate bowl, combine the rest of the soup with the almond flour, dry mustard, ketchup, Worcestershire sauce, and ¼ cup water. Pour this over the beef meatballs, cover the pan, and cook for 10 minutes as you stir occasionally. Split among bowls and serve.

Nutrition:

Kcal 332

Fat 18g

Net Carbs 7g

Protein 25g

Beef & Ale Pot Roast

Preparation Time: 30 minutes

Cooking Time: 2 hours 20 minutes

Servings: 6

Ingredients:

- 1 ½ lb. brisket
- 2 tbsp olive oil
- 8 baby carrots, peeled
- 2 medium red onions, quartered
- 1 celery stalk, cut into chunks
- Salt and black pepper to taste
- 2 bay leaves
- 1 ½ cups low carb beer (ale)

Directions:

1. Preheat oven to 370ºF. Heat the olive oil in a large skillet over medium heat. Season the brisket with salt and pepper.

2. Brown the meat on both sides for 8 minutes. After, transfer to a deep casserole dish. In the dish, arrange the

carrots, onions, celery, and bay leaves around the brisket and pour the beer all over it.

3. Cover the pot and cook in the oven for 2 hours. When ready, remove the casserole. Transfer the beef to a chopping board and cut it into thick slices. Serve the beef and vegetables with a drizzle of the sauce.

Nutrition:
Calories: 302.2
Fat: 22.7g
Carb: 9.3g,
Protein: 8g

Beef Tripe Pot

Preparation Time: 10 minutes
Cooking Time: 1 hour 30 minutes
Servings: 6
Ingredients:

- 1 ½ lb. beef tripe, cleaned
- 4 cups buttermilk
- Salt and black pepper to taste
- 3 tbsp olive oil
- 2 onions, sliced
- 4 garlic cloves, minced
- 3 tomatoes, diced
- 1 tsp paprika
- 2 chili peppers, minced

Directions:

1. Put the tripe in a bowl and cover with buttermilk. Refrigerate for 3 hours to extract bitterness and gamey taste.
2. Remove from buttermilk, drain and rinse well under cold running water. Place in a pot over medium heat and cover with water. Bring to a boil and cook about for 1 hour until tender.

Remove the tripe with a perforated spoon and let cool. Strain the broth and reserve. Chop the cooled tripe.

3. Heat the oil in a skillet over medium heat. Sauté the onions, garlic, and chili peppers for 3 minutes until soft. Stir in the paprika and add in the tripe. Cook for 5-6 minutes. Include the tomatoes and 4 cups of the reserved tripe broth and cook for 10 minutes. Adjust the seasoning with salt and pepper. Serve.

Nutrition:
Kcal 248
Fat 12.8g
Net Carbs 4g
Protein 8g

Beef Stovies

Preparation Time: 12 minutes
Cooking Time: 45 minutes
Servings: 4
Ingredients:

- 1 lb. ground beef
- 1 large onion, chopped
- 2 parsnips, peeled and chopped
- 1 large carrot, chopped
- 2 tbsp olive oil
- 2 garlic cloves, minced
- Salt and black pepper to taste
- 1 cup chicken broth
- ¼ tsp allspice
- 2 tsp fresh rosemary, chopped
- 1 tbsp Worcestershire sauce
- ½ small cabbage, shredded

Directions:

1. Heat the olive oil in a skillet over medium heat and cook the beef for 4

minutes. Season with salt and pepper, stirring occasionally while breaking the lumps in it.

2. Add in onion, garlic, carrot, rosemary, and parsnips.
3. Stir and cook for a minute, and pour in the chicken broth, allspice, and Worcestershire sauce.
4. Reduce the heat to low and cook for 20 minutes. Stir in the cabbage, season with salt and black pepper, and cook further for 15 minutes. Turn the heat off, plate the stovies, and serve warm.

Nutrition:

Kcal 316

Fat 18g

Net Carbs 3g

Protein 14g

Beef and Sausage Medley

Preparation Time: 10 minutes

Cooking Time: 27 minutes

Servings: 8

Ingredients:

- 1 teaspoon butter
- 2 beef sausages, casing removed and sliced
- 2 pounds (907 g) beef steak, cubed
- 1 yellow onion, sliced
- 2 fresh ripe tomatoes, puréed
- 1 jalapeño pepper, chopped
- 1 red bell pepper, chopped
- 1½ cups roasted vegetable broth
- 2 cloves garlic, minced
- 1 teaspoon Old Bay seasoning
- 2 bay leaves
- 1 sprig thyme
- 1 sprig rosemary

- ½ teaspoon paprika
- Sea salt and ground black pepper, to taste

Directions:

1. Press the Sauté button to heat up the Instant Pot. Melt the butter and cook the sausage and steak for 4 minutes, stirring periodically. Set aside.
2. Add the onion and sauté for 3 minutes or until softened and translucent. Add the remaining ingredients, including reserved beef and sausage.
3. Secure the lid. Choose Manual mode and set time for 20 minutes on High Pressure.
4. Once cooking is complete, use a quick pressure release. Carefully remove the lid.
5. Serve immediately.

Nutrition:

Calories: 319

Fat: 14.0g

Protein: 42.8g

Carbs: 6.3g

Net carbs: 1.8g

Fiber: 4.5g

Beef Back Ribs with Barbecue Glaze

Preparation Time: 10 minutes

Cooking Time: 35 minutes

Servings: 4

Ingredients:

- ½ cup water

- 1 (3-pound / 1.4-kg) rack beef back ribs, prepared with rub of choice
- ¼ cup unsweetened tomato purée
- ¼ teaspoon Worcestershire sauce
- ¼ teaspoon garlic powder
- 2 teaspoons apple cider vinegar
- ¼ teaspoon liquid smoke
- ¼ teaspoon smoked paprika
- 3 tablespoons Swerve
- Dash of cayenne pepper

Directions:

1. Pour the water in the pot and place the trivet inside.
2. Arrange the ribs on top of the trivet.
3. Close the lid. Select Manual mode and set cooking time for 25 minutes on High Pressure.
4. Meanwhile, prepare the glaze by whisking together the tomato purée, Worcestershire sauce, garlic powder, vinegar, liquid smoke, paprika, Swerve, and cayenne in a medium bowl. Heat the broiler.
5. When timer beeps, quick release the pressure. Open the lid. Remove the ribs and place on a baking sheet.
6. Brush a layer of glaze on the ribs. Put under the broiler for 5 minutes.
7. Remove from the broiler and brush with glaze again. Put back under the broiler for 5 more minutes, or until the tops are sticky.
8. Serve immediately.

Nutrition:

Calories: 758

Fat: 26.8g

Protein: 33.7g

Carbs: 0.9g

Net carbs: 0.7g

Fiber: 0.2g

Beef Big Mac Salad

Preparation Time: 10 minutes

Cooking Time: 9 minutes

Servings: 2

Ingredients:

- 5 ounces (142 g) ground beef
- 1 teaspoon ground black pepper
- 1 tablespoon sesame oil
- 1 cup lettuce, chopped
- ¼ cup Monterey Jack cheese, shredded
- 2 ounces (57 g) dill pickles, sliced
- 1 ounce (28 g) scallions, chopped
- 1 tablespoon heavy cream

Directions:

1. In a mixing bowl, combine the ground beef and ground black pepper. Shape the mixture into mini burgers.
2. Pour the sesame oil in the Instant Pot and heat for 3 minutes on Sauté mode.
3. Place the mini hamburgers in the hot oil and cook for 3 minutes on each side.
4. Meanwhile, in a salad bowl, mix the chopped lettuce, shredded cheese, dill pickles, scallions, and heavy cream. Toss to mix well.

5. Top the salad with cooked mini burgers. Serve immediately.

Nutrition:

Calories: 284

Fat: 18.5g

Protein: 25.7g

Carbs: 3.5g

Net carbs: 2.3g

Fiber: 1.2g

Beef Bourguignon

Preparation Time: 15 minutes

Cooking Time: 35 minutes

Servings: 6

Ingredients:

- 3 ounces (85 g) bacon, chopped
- 1 pound (454 g) beef tenderloin, chopped
- ¼ cup apple cider vinegar
- ¼ teaspoon ground coriander
- ¼ teaspoon xanthan gum
- 1 teaspoon dried oregano
- 1 teaspoon unsweetened tomato purée
- 1 cup beef broth

Directions:

1. Put the bacon in the Instant Pot and cook for 5 minutes on Sauté mode. Flip the bacon with a spatula every 1 minute.
2. Add the chopped beef tenderloin, apple cider vinegar, ground coriander, xanthan gum, and dried oregano.

3. Add the tomato purée and beef broth. Stir to mix well and close the lid.
4. Select Manual mode and set cooking time for 30 minutes on High Pressure.
5. When timer beeps, make a quick pressure release. Open the lid.
6. Serve immediately.

Nutrition:

Calories: 245

Fat: 13.1g

Protein: 28.0g

Carbs: 1.3g

Net carbs: 0.6g

Fiber: 0.7g

Beef Brisket with Cabbage

Preparation Time: 15 minutes

Cooking Time: 1 hour 7 minutes

Servings: 8

Ingredients:

- 3 pounds (1.4 kg) corned beef brisket
- 4 cups water
- 3 garlic cloves, minced
- 2 teaspoons yellow mustard seed
- 2 teaspoons black peppercorns
- 3 celery stalks, chopped
- ½ large white onion, chopped
- 1 green cabbage, cut into quarters

Directions:

1. Add the brisket to the Instant Pot. Pour the water into the pot. Add the garlic, mustard seed, and black peppercorns.
2. Lock the lid. Select Meat/Stew mode and set

cooking time for 50 minutes on High Pressure.

3. When cooking is complete, allow the pressure to release naturally for 20 minutes, then release any remaining pressure. Open the lid and transfer only the brisket to a platter.
4. Add the celery, onion, and cabbage to the pot.
5. Lock the lid. Select Soup mode and set cooking time for 12 minutes on High Pressure.
6. When cooking is complete, quick release the pressure. Open the lid, add the brisket back to the pot and let warm in the pot for 5 minutes.
7. Transfer the warmed brisket back to the platter and thinly slice. Transfer the vegetables to the platter. Serve hot.

Nutrition:

Calories: 357 Fat: 25.5g
Protein: 26.3g Carbs: 7.3g
Net carbs: 5.3g Fiber: 2.0g

Beef Carne Guisada

Preparation Time: 10 minutes

Cooking Time: 20 minutes

Servings: 4

Ingredients:

- 2 tomatoes, chopped
- 1 red bell pepper, chopped
- ½ onion, chopped
- 3 garlic cloves, chopped
- 1 teaspoon ancho chili powder

- 1 tablespoon ground cumin
- ½ teaspoon dried oregano
- 1 teaspoons salt
- 1 teaspoon freshly ground black pepper
- 1 teaspoon smoked paprika
- 1 pound (454 g) beef chuck, cut into large pieces
- ¾ cup water, plus 2 tablespoons
- ¼ teaspoon xanthan gum

Directions:

1. In a blender, purée the tomatoes, bell pepper, onion, garlic, chili powder, cumin, oregano, salt, pepper, and paprika.
2. Put the beef pieces in the Instant Pot. Pour in the blended mixture.
3. Use ¾ cup of water to wash out the blender and pour the liquid into the pot.
4. Lock the lid. Select Manual mode and set cooking time for 20 minutes on High Pressure.
5. When cooking is complete, quick release the pressure. Unlock the lid.
6. Switch the pot to Sauté mode. Bring the stew to a boil.
7. Put the xanthan gum and 2 tablespoons of water into the boiling stew and stir until it thickens.
8. Serve immediately.

Nutrition:

Calories: 326 Fat: 22.0g
Protein: 23.0g Carbs: 9.0g
Net carbs: 7.0g Fiber: 2.0g

CHAPTER 7:

Pork Recipes

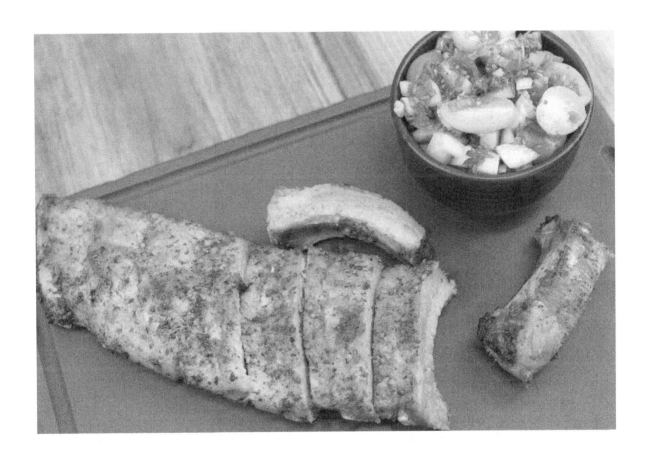

Cilantro Garlic Pork Chops

Preparation Time: 10 Minutes

Cooking Time: 15 Minutes

Servings: 4

Ingredients:

- 1 pound boneless center-cut pork chops, pounded to ¼ inch thick
- Sea salt, for seasoning
- Freshly ground black pepper, for seasoning
- ¼ cup good-quality olive oil, divided
- ¼ cup finely chopped fresh cilantro
- 1 tablespoon minced garlic
- Juice of 1 lime

Directions:

1. Marinate the pork. Pat the pork chops dry and season them lightly with salt and pepper. Place them in a large bowl, add 2 tablespoons of the olive oil, and the cilantro, garlic, and lime juice. Toss to coat the chops. Cover the bowl and marinate the chops at room temperature for 30 minutes. Cook the pork. In a large skillet over medium-high heat, warm the remaining 2 tablespoons of olive oil. Add the pork chops in a single layer and fry them, turning them once, until they're just cooked through and still juicy, 6 to 7 minutes per side.

2.
   Serve. Divide the chops between four plates and serve them immediately.

Nutrition:

Calories: 249

Total fat: 16g

Total carbs: 2g

Fiber: 0g;

Net carbs: 2g

Sodium: 261mg

Protein: 25g

Spinach Feta Stuffed Pork

Preparation Time: 15 Minutes

Cooking Time: 30 Minutes

Servings: 4

Ingredients:

- 4 ounces crumbled feta cheese
- ¾ cup chopped frozen spinach, thawed and liquid squeezed out
- 3 tablespoons chopped Kalamata olives
- 4 (4-ounce) center pork chops, 2 inches thick
- Sea salt, for seasoning
- Freshly ground black pepper, for seasoning
- 3 tablespoons good-quality olive oil

Directions:

1. Preheat the oven. Set the oven temperature to 400°F.
2. Make the filling. In a small bowl, mix together the feta, spinach, and olives until everything is well combined.
3. Stuff the pork chops. Make a horizontal slit in the side of each chop to create a pocket, making sure you don't cut all the way through. Stuff the filling equally between the chops and secure the slits with toothpicks. Lightly season the stuffed chops with salt and pepper.
4. Brown the chops. In a large oven-safe skillet over medium-high heat, warm the olive oil.

5. Add the chops and sear them until they're browned all over, about 10 minutes in total.
6. Roast the chops. Place the skillet in the oven and roast the chops for 20 minutes or until they're cooked through.
7. Serve. Let the meat rest for 10 minutes and then remove the toothpicks. Divide the pork chops between four plates and serve them immediately.

Nutrition:

Calories: 342

Total fat: 24g

Total carbs: 3g

Fiber: 1g;

Net carbs: 2g

Sodium: 572mg

Protein: 28g

Coconut Milk Ginger Marinated Pork Tenderloin

Preparation Time: 5 Minutes

Cooking Time: 25 Minutes

Servings: 4

Ingredients:

- ¼ cup coconut oil, divided
- 1½ pounds boneless pork chops, about ¾ inch thick
- 1 tablespoon grated fresh ginger
- 2 teaspoons minced garlic
- 1 cup coconut milk
- 1 teaspoon chopped fresh basil
- Juice of 1 lime
- ½ cup shredded unsweetened coconut

Directions:

1. Brown the pork. In a large skillet over medium heat, warm 2 tablespoons of the coconut oil. Add the pork chops to the skillet and brown them all over, turning them several times, about 10 minutes in total.
2. Braise the pork. Move the pork to the side of the skillet and add the remaining 2 tablespoons of coconut oil. Add the ginger and garlic and sauté until they've softened, about 2 minutes. Stir in the coconut milk, basil, and lime juice and move the pork back to the center of the skillet. Cover the skillet and simmer until the pork is just cooked through and very tender, 12 to 15 minutes.
3. Serve. Divide the pork chops between four plates and top them with the shredded coconut.

Nutrition:

Calories: 479

Total fat: 38g

Total carbs: 6g

Fiber: 3g;

Net carbs: 3g

Sodium: 318mg

Protein: 32g

Grilled Pork Chops with Greek Salsa

Preparation Time: 15 Minutes

Cooking Time: 15 Minutes

Servings: 4

Ingredients:

- ¼ cup good-quality olive oil, divided
- 1 tablespoon red wine vinegar

- 3 teaspoons chopped fresh oregano, divided
- 1 teaspoon minced garlic
- 4 (4-ounce) boneless center-cut loin pork chops
- ½ cup halved cherry tomatoes
- ½ yellow bell pepper, diced
- ½ English cucumber, chopped
- ¼ red onion, chopped
- 1 tablespoon balsamic vinegar
- Sea salt, for seasoning
- Freshly ground black pepper, for seasoning

Directions:

1. Marinate the pork. In a medium bowl, stir together 3 tablespoons of the olive oil, the vinegar, 2 teaspoons of the oregano, and the garlic. Add the pork chops to the bowl, turning them to get them coated with the marinade. Cover the bowl and place it in the refrigerator for 30 minutes.
2. Make the salsa. While the pork is marinating, in a medium bowl, stir together the remaining 1 tablespoon of olive oil, the tomatoes, yellow bell pepper, cucumber, red onion, vinegar, and the remaining 1 teaspoon of oregano. Season the salsa with salt and pepper. Set the bowl aside.
3. Grill the pork chops. Heat a grill to medium-high heat. Remove the pork chops from the marinade and grill them until just cooked through, 6 to 8 minutes per side.
4. Serve. Rest the pork for 5 minutes. Divide the pork between four plates and serve them with a generous scoop of the salsa.

Nutrition:

Calories: 277

Total fat: 19g

Total carbs: 4g

Fiber: 1g;

Net carbs: 3g

Sodium: 257mg; Protein: 25g

Grilled Herbed Pork Kebabs

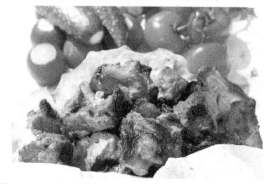

Preparation Time: 10 Minutes

Cooking Time: 15 Minutes

Servings: 4

Ingredients:

- ¼ cup good-quality olive oil
- 1 tablespoon minced garlic
- 2 teaspoons dried oregano
- 1 teaspoon dried basil
- 1 teaspoon dried parsley
- ½ teaspoon sea salt
- 1/4 teaspoon freshly ground black pepper
- 1 (1-pound) pork tenderloin, cut into 1½-inch pieces

Directions:

1. Marinate the pork. In a medium bowl, stir together the olive oil, garlic, oregano, basil, parsley, salt, and pepper. Add the pork pieces and toss

to coat them in the marinade. Cover the bowl and place it in the refrigerator for 2 to 4 hours.

2. Make the kebabs. Divide the pork pieces between four skewers, making sure not to crowd the meat.

3. Grill the kebabs. Preheat your grill to medium-high heat. Grill the skewers for about 12 minutes, turning to cook all sides of the pork, until the pork is cooked through.

4. Serve. Rest the skewers for 5 minutes. Divide the skewers between four plates and serve them immediately.

Nutrition:

Calories: 261

Total fat: 18g

Total carbs: 1g

Fiber: 0g;

Net carbs: 1g

Sodium: 60mg

Protein: 24

Italian Sausage Broccoli Sauté

Preparation Time: 10 Minutes

Cooking Time: 20 Minutes

Servings: 4

Ingredients:

- 2 tablespoons good-quality olive oil
- 1 pound Italian sausage meat, hot or mild
- 4 cups small broccoli florets
- 1 tablespoon minced garlic
- Freshly ground black pepper, for seasoning

Directions:

1. Cook the sausage. In a large skillet over medium heat, warm the olive oil. Add the sausage and sauté it until it's cooked through, 8 to 10 minutes. Transfer the sausage to a plate with a slotted spoon and set the plate aside.

2. Sauté the vegetables. Add the broccoli to the skillet and sauté it until its tender, about 6 minutes. Stir in the garlic and sauté for another 3 minutes.

3. Finish the dish. Return the sausage to the skillet and toss to combine it with the other ingredients. Season the mixture with pepper.

4. Serve. Divide the mixture between four plates and serve it immediately.

Nutrition:

Calories: 486

Total fat: 43g

Total carbs: 7g

Fiber: 2g;

Net carbs: 5g

Sodium: 513mg

Protein: 19g

Classic Sausage and Peppers

Preparation Time: 10 Minutes

Cooking Time: 35 Minutes

Servings: 6

Ingredients:

- 1½ pounds sweet Italian sausages (or hot if you prefer)
- 2 tablespoons good-quality olive oil
- 1 red bell pepper, cut into thin strips
- 1 yellow bell pepper, cut into thin strips

- 1 orange bell pepper, cut into thin strips
- 1 red onion, thinly sliced
- 1 tablespoon minced garlic
- ½ cup white wine
- Sea salt, for seasoning
- Freshly ground black pepper, for seasoning

Directions:

1. Cook the sausage. Preheat a grill to medium-high and grill the sausages, turning them several times, until they're cooked through, about 12 minutes in total. Let the sausages rest for 15 minutes and then cut them into 2-inch pieces.
2. Sauté the vegetables. In a large skillet over medium-high heat, warm the olive oil. Add the red, yellow, and orange bell peppers, and the red onion and garlic and sauté until they're tender, about 10 minutes.
3. Finish the dish. Add the sausage to the skillet along with the white wine and sauté for 10 minutes.
4. Serve. Divide the mixture between four plates, season it with salt and pepper, and serve.

Nutrition:

Calories: 450

Total fat: 40g

Total carbs: 5g

Fiber: 1g;

Net carbs: 4g

Sodium: 554mg

Protein: 17g

Lemon-Infused Pork Rib Roast

Preparation Time: 10 Minutes

Cooking Time: 1 Hour

Servings: 6

Ingredients:

- ¼ cup good-quality olive oil
- Zest and juice of 1 lemon
- Zest and juice of 1 orange
- 4 rosemary sprigs, lightly crushed
- 4 thyme sprigs, lightly crushed
- 1 (4-bone) pork rib roast, about 2½ pounds
- 6 garlic cloves, peeled
- Sea salt, for seasoning
- Freshly ground black pepper, for seasoning

Directions:

1. Make the marinade. In a large bowl, combine the olive oil, lemon zest, lemon juice, orange zest, orange juice, rosemary sprigs, and thyme sprigs.
2. Marinate the roast. Use a small knife to make six 1-inch-deep slits in the fatty side of the roast. Stuff the garlic cloves in the slits. Put the roast in the bowl with the marinade and turn it to coat it well with the marinade. Cover the bowl and refrigerate it overnight, turning the roast in the marinade several times.
3. Preheat the oven. Set the oven temperature to 350°F.
4. Roast the pork. Remove the pork from the marinade and season it with salt and pepper, then put it in a baking dish and let it come to room temperature. Roast the pork until it's cooked through (145°F to 160°F internal temperature), about 1 hour. Throw out any leftover marinade.

5. Serve. Let the pork rest for 10 minutes, then cut it into slices and arrange the slices on a platter. Serve it warm.

Nutrition:

Calories: 403

Total fat: 30g

Total carbs: 1g

Fiber: 0g;

Net carbs: 1g

Sodium: 113mg

Protein: 30g

Pork Meatball Parmesan

Preparation Time: 15 Minutes

Cooking Time: 30 Minutes

Servings: 6

Ingredients:

For The Meatballs:

- 1¼ Pounds ground pork
- ½ cup almond flour
- ½ cup Parmesan cheese
- 1 egg, lightly beaten
- 1 tablespoon chopped fresh parsley
- 1 teaspoon minced garlic
- 1 teaspoon chopped fresh oregano
- ¼ teaspoon sea salt
- 1/8 teaspoon freshly ground black pepper
- 2 tablespoons good-quality olive oil

FOR THE PARMIGIANA:

- 1 cup sugar-free tomato sauce
- 1 cup shredded mozzarella cheese

Directions:

1. Make the meatballs. In a large bowl, mix together the ground pork, almond flour, Parmesan, egg, parsley, garlic, oregano, salt, and pepper until everything is well mixed. Roll the pork mixture into 1½-inch meatballs.

2. Cook the meatballs. In a large skillet over medium-high heat, warm the olive oil. Add the meatballs to the skillet and cook them, turning them several times, until they're thoroughly cooked through, about 15 minutes in total.

TO MAKE THE PARMIGIANA:

3. Preheat the oven. Set the oven temperature to 350°F.

4. Assemble the parmigiana. Transfer the meatballs to a 9-by-9-inch baking dish and top them with the tomato sauce. Sprinkle with the mozzarella and bake for 15 minutes or until the cheese is melted and golden.

5. Serve. Divide the meatballs and sauce between six bowls and serve it immediately.

Nutrition:

Calories: 403

Total fat: 32g

Total carbs: 1g

Fiber: 0g;

Net carbs: 1g

Sodium: 351mg

Protein: 25g

CHAPTER 8:

Lamb Recipes

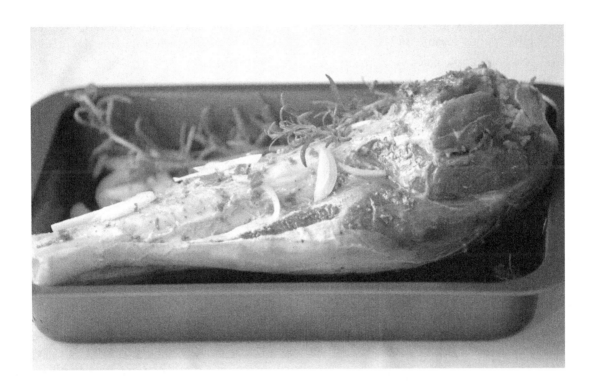

Chipotle Lamb Ribs

Preparation Time: 15 minutes

Cooking Time: 20 minutes

Servings: 6

Ingredients:

- 2-pound lamb ribs
- 1 tablespoon chipotle pepper, minced
- 2 tablespoons sesame oil
- 1 teaspoon apple cider vinegar

Directions:

1. Mix lamb ribs with all ingredients and leave to marinate for 10 minutes.
2. Then transfer the lamb ribs and all marinade in the baking tray and cook the meat in the oven at 360F for 40 minutes. Flip the ribs on another side after 20 minutes of cooking.

Nutrition:

Calories 392 Fat 24.7

Fiber 0

Carbs 0.2

Protein 39.6

Lamb and Pecan Salad

Preparation Time: 10 minutes

Cooking Time: 10 minutes

Servings: 4

Ingredients:

- 2 lamb chops
- 1 tablespoon sesame oil
- 2 pecans, chopped
- 2 cups lettuce, chopped
- 1 teaspoon cayenne pepper
- 1 tablespoon avocado oil

Directions:

1. Sprinkle the lamb chops with cayenne pepper and put in the hot skillet.
2. Add sesame oil and roast the meat for 4 minutes per side.
3. Then chops the lamb chops and put them in the salad bowl.
4. Add all remaining ingredients and carefully mix the salad.

Nutrition:

Calories 168

Fat 12.1

Fiber 1

Carbs 2.3

Protein 12.9

Hot Sauce Lamb

Preparation Time: 10 minutes

Cooking Time: 35 minutes

Servings: 4

Ingredients:

- 2 teaspoons paprika
- 1-pound lamb fillet, chopped
- 1 tablespoon coconut oil
- 4 tablespoons keto hot sauce
- ½ cup of water

Directions:

1. Pour water in the saucepan and bring it to boil.
2. Add lamb and boil it for 20 minutes.
3. After this, preheat the skillet well.
4. Add boiled lamb fillet, coconut oil, and paprika.
5. Roast the ingredients for 6 minutes per side or until the meat is light brown.

6. Then add hot sauce and carefully mix the meal.

Nutrition:

Calories 245

Fat 11.9

Fiber 0.4

Carbs 0.8

Protein 32.1

Mustard Lamb Chops

Preparation Time: 10 minutes

Cooking Time: 40 minutes

Servings: 4

Ingredients:

- 1 cup spinach
- 3 tablespoons mustard
- 2 tablespoons sesame oil
- ½ teaspoon ground turmeric
- 4 lamb chops

Directions:

1. Blend the spinach and mix it with mustard, sesame oil, and ground turmeric.
2. Then rub the lamb chops with the mustard mixture and put in the baking pan.
3. Bake the meat at 355F for 40 minutes. Flip the meat after 20 minutes of cooking.

Nutrition:

Calories 102

Fat 9.3

Fiber 1.5

Carbs 3.4

Protein 2.3

Ginger Lamb Chops

Preparation Time: 15 minutes

Cooking Time: 30 minutes

Servings: 6

Ingredients:

- 6 lamb chops
- 1 tablespoon keto tomato paste
- 1 teaspoon minced ginger
- 2 tablespoons avocado oil
- 1 teaspoon plain yogurt

Directions:

1. Mix plain yogurt with keto tomato paste and minced ginger.
2. Then put the lamb chops in the yogurt mixture and marinate for 10-15 minutes.
3. After this, transfer the mixture in the tray, add avocado oil, and cook the meat at 360F in the oven for 30 minutes.

Nutrition:

Calories 330

Fat 26.6

Fiber 0.4

Carbs 1

Protein 19.3

Parmesan Lamb

Preparation Time: 10 minutes

Cooking Time: 20 minutes

Servings: 4

Ingredients:

- 4 lamb chops
- 2 oz. Parmesan, grated
- ½ cup plain yogurt
- 3 scallions, sliced
- 1 tablespoon butter, softened

Directions:

1. Melt the butter in the saucepan. Add scallions and roast it for 3-4 minutes.
2. Then stir the scallions and add lamb chops.
3. Roast them for 2 minutes per side.
4. Add yogurt and close the lid. Cook the meat for 10 minutes.
5. After this, top the meat with Parmesan and cook it for 2 minutes more.

Nutrition:

Calories 262

Fat 12.6

Fiber 0.6

Carbs 5.2

Protein 30.5

Clove Lamb

Preparation Time: 10 minutes

Cooking Time: 25 minutes

Servings: 4

Ingredients:

- 1 teaspoon ground clove
- 2 tablespoons butter
- 1 teaspoon ground paprika
- 1 teaspoon dried rosemary
- ¼ cup of water
- 12 oz. lamb fillet

Directions:

1. In the shallow bowl, mix ground clove with ground paprika, and dried rosemary.
2. Rub the lamb fillet with spices and grease with butter.

3. Then put the meat in the hot skillet and roast it for 5 minutes per side on the low heat.
4. Add water. Close the lid and cook the lamb on medium heat for 15 minutes.

Nutrition:

Calories 55

Fat 6

Fiber 0.5

Carbs 0.8

Protein 0.2

Carrot Lamb Roast

Preparation Time: 10 minutes

Cooking Time: 40 minutes

Servings: 4

Ingredients:

- 1-pound lamb loin
- 1 carrot, chopped
- 1 teaspoon dried thyme
- 2 tablespoons coconut oil
- 1 teaspoon salt

Directions:

1. Put all ingredients in the baking tray, mix well.
2. Bake the mixture in the preheated to 360F oven for 40 minutes.

Nutrition:

Calories 295

Fat 17.9

Fiber 0.5

Carbs 1.7

Protein 30.3

Lamb and Celery Casserole

Preparation Time: 10 minutes

Cooking Time: 45 minutes

Servings: 2

Ingredients:

- ¼ cup celery stalk, chopped
- 2 lamb chops, chopped
- ½ cup Mozzarella, shredded
- 1 teaspoon butter
- ¼ cup coconut cream
- 1 teaspoon taco seasonings

Directions:

1. Mix lamb chops with taco seasonings and put in the casserole mold.
2. Add celery stalk, coconut cream, and shredded mozzarella.
3. Then add butter and cook the casserole in the preheated to 360F oven for 45 minutes.

Nutrition:

Calories 283

Fat 19.3

Fiber 0.9

Carbs 3.3

Protein 24.8

Lamb in Almond Sauce

Preparation Time: 10 minutes

Cooking Time: 30 minutes

Servings: 6

Ingredients:

- 14 oz. lamb fillet, cubed
- 1 cup organic almond milk
- 1 teaspoon almond flour
- 1 teaspoon ground nutmeg
- ½ teaspoon ground cardamom

- 1 tablespoon olive oil
- 1 tablespoon lemon juice
- 1 tablespoon butter
- ½ teaspoon minced garlic

Directions:

1. Preheat the olive oil in the saucepan.
2. Meanwhile, mix lamb, ground nutmeg, ground cardamom, and minced garlic.
3. Put the lamb in the hot olive oil. Roast the meat for 2 minutes per side.
4. Then add butter, lemon juice, and almond milk. Carefully mix the mixture.
5. Cook the meal for 15 minutes on medium heat.
6. Then add almond flour, stir well and simmer the meal for 10 minutes more.

Nutrition:

Calories 258

Fat 19

Fiber 1.1

Carbs 2.7

Protein 19.7

Sweet Leg of Lamb

Preparation Time: 10 minutes

Cooking Time: 45 minutes

Servings: 6

Ingredients:

- 2 pounds lamb leg
- 1 tablespoon Erythritol
- 3 tablespoons coconut milk
- 1 teaspoon chili flakes
- 1 teaspoon ground turmeric

- 1 teaspoon cayenne pepper
- 3 tablespoons coconut oil

Directions:

1. In the shallow bowl, mix cayenne pepper, ground turmeric, chili flakes, and Erythritol.
2. Rub the lamb leg with spices.
3. Melt the coconut oil in the saucepan.
4. Add lamb leg and roast it for 10 minutes per side on low heat.
5. After this, add coconut milk and cook the meal for 30 minutes on low heat. Flip the meat on another side from time to time.

Nutrition:

Calories 350

Fat 18.8

Fiber 0.3

Carbs 0.8

Protein 42.8

Coconut Lamb Shoulder

Preparation Time: 10 minutes

Cooking Time: 75 minutes

Servings: 5

Ingredients:

- 2-pound lamb shoulder
- 1 teaspoon ground cumin
- 2 tablespoons butter
- ¼ cup of coconut milk
- 1 teaspoon coconut shred
- ½ cup kale, chopped

Directions:

1. Put all ingredients in the saucepan and mix well.
2. Close the lid and cook the meal on low heat for 75 minutes.

Nutrition:

Calories 414

Fat 21.2

Fiber 0.5

Carbs 1.7

Protein 51.5

Lavender Lamb

Preparation Time: 10 minutes

Cooking Time: 35 minutes

Servings: 4

Ingredients:

- 4 lamb chops
- 1 teaspoon dried lavender
- 2 tablespoons butter
- 1 teaspoon cumin seeds
- 1 cup of water

Directions:

1. Toss the butter in the saucepan and melt it.
2. Add lamb chops and roast them for 3 minutes.
3. Then add dried lavender, cumin seeds, and water.
4. Close the lid and cook the meat for 30 minutes on medium-low heat.

Nutrition:

Calories 211

Fat 12.1

Fiber 0.1

Carbs 0.2

Protein 24

Dill Lamb Shank

Preparation Time: 10 minutes
Cooking Time: 40 minutes
Servings: 3
Ingredients:

- 3 lamb shanks (4 oz. each)
- 1 tablespoon dried dill
- 1 teaspoon peppercorns
- 3 cups of water
- 1 carrot, chopped
- 1 teaspoon salt

Directions:

1. Bring the water to boil.
2. Add lamb shank, dried dill, peppercorns, carrot, and salt.
3. Close the lid and cook the meat in medium heat for 40 minutes.

Nutrition:

Calories 224

Fat 84

Fiber 0.8

Carbs 3

Protein 32.3

Mexican Lamb Chops

Preparation Time: 10 minutes
Cooking Time: 15 minutes
Servings: 4
Ingredients:

- 4 lamb chops
- 1 tablespoon Mexican seasonings
- 2 tablespoons sesame oil
- 1 teaspoon butter

Directions:

1. Rub the lamb chops with Mexican seasonings.
2. Then melt the butter in the skillet. Add sesame oil.
3. Then add lamb chops and roast them for 7 minutes per side on medium heat.

Nutrition:

Calories 323

Fat 14

Fiber 0

Carbs 1.1

Protein 24.1

CHAPTER 9:

Seafood

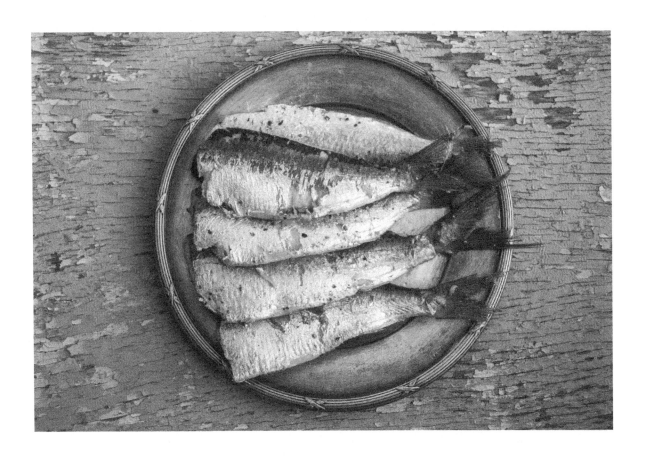

Fish and Egg Plate

Preparation Time: 5 minutes;

Cooking Time: 10 minutes;

Servings: 2

Ingredients

- 2 eggs
- 1 tbsp. butter, unsalted
- 2 pacific whitening fillets
- ½ oz. chopped lettuce
- 1 scallion, chopped
- Seasoning:
- 3 tbsp. avocado oil
- 1/3 tsp salt
- 1/3 tsp ground black pepper

Directions:

1. Cook the eggs and for this, take a frying pan, place it over medium heat, add butter and when it melts, crack the egg in the pan and cook for 2 to 3 minutes until fried to desired liking.
2. Transfer fried egg to a plate and then cook the remaining egg in the same manner.
3. Meanwhile, season fish fillets with ¼ tsp each of salt and black pepper.
4. When eggs have fried, sprinkle salt and black pepper on them, then add 1 tbsp. oil into the frying pan, add fillets and cook for 4 minutes per side until thoroughly cooked.
5. When done, distribute fillets to the plate, add lettuce and scallion, drizzle with remaining oil, and then serve.

Sesame Tuna Salad

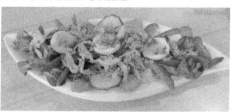

Preparation Time: 35 minutes

Cooking Time: 0 minutes;

Servings: 2

Ingredients

- 6 oz. of tuna in water
- ½ tbsp. chili-garlic paste
- ½ tbsp. black sesame seeds, toasted
- 2 tbsp. mayonnaise
- 1 tbsp. sesame oil
- Seasoning:
- 1/8 tsp red pepper flakes

Directions:

1. Take a medium bowl, all the ingredients for the salad in it except for tuna, and then stir until well combined.
2. Fold in tuna until mixed and then refrigerator for 30 minutes.
3. Serve.

Nutrition: 322 Calories; 25.4 g Fats; 17.7 g Protein; 2.6 g Net Carb; 3 g Fiber;

Keto Tuna Sandwich

Preparation Time: 10 minutes

Cooking Time: 10 minutes;

Servings: 2

Ingredients

- 2 oz. tuna, packed in water
- 2 2/3 tbsp. coconut flour
- 1 tsp baking powder
- 2 eggs

- 2 tbsp. mayonnaise
- Seasoning:
- 1/4 tsp salt
- 1/4 tsp ground black pepper

Directions:

1. Turn on the oven, then set it to 375 degrees F and let it preheat.
2. Meanwhile, prepare the batter for this, add all the ingredients in a bowl, reserving mayonnaise, 1 egg, and 1/8 tsp salt, and then whisk until well combined.
3. Take a 4 by 4 inches heatproof baking pan, grease it with oil, pour in the prepared batter and bake 10 minutes until bread is firm.
4. Meanwhile, prepare tuna and for this, place tuna in a medium bowl, add mayonnaise, season with remaining salt and black pepper, and then stir until combined.
5. When done, let the bread cool in the pan for 5 minutes, then transfer it to a wire rack and cool for 20 minutes.
6. Slice the bread, prepare sandwiches with prepared tuna mixture, and then serve.

Nutrition: 255 Calories; 17.8 g Fats; 16.3 g Protein; 3.7 g Net Carb; 3.3 g Fiber;

Tuna Melt Jalapeno Peppers

Preparation Time: 5 minutes

Cooking Time: 10 minutes;

Servings: 2

Ingredients

- 4 jalapeno peppers
- 1-ounce tuna, packed in water
- 1-ounce cream cheese softened
- 1 tbsp. grated parmesan cheese

- 1 tbsp. grated mozzarella cheese
- Seasoning:
- 1 tsp chopped dill pickles
- 1 green onion, green part sliced only

Directions:

1. Turn on the oven, then set it to 400 degrees F and let it preheat.
2. Prepare the peppers and for this, cut each pepper in half lengthwise and remove seeds and stem.
3. Take a small bowl, place tuna in it, add remaining ingredients except for cheeses, and then stir until combined.
4. Spoon tuna mixture into peppers, sprinkle cheeses on top, and then bake for 7 to 10 minutes until cheese has turned golden brown.
5. Serve.

Nutrition: 104 Calories; 6.2 g Fats; 7 g Protein; 2.1 g Net Carb; 1.1 g Fiber;

Smoked Salmon Fat Bombs

Preparation Time: 5 minutes

Cooking Time: 0 minutes;

Servings: 2

Ingredients

- 2 tbsp. cream cheese, softened
- 1 ounce smoked salmon
- 2 tsp bagel seasoning

Directions:

1. Take a medium bowl, place cream cheese and salmon in it, and stir until well combined.
2. Shape the mixture into bowls, roll them into bagel seasoning and then serve.

Nutrition: 65 Calories; 4.8 g Fats; 4 g Protein; 0.5 g Net Carb; 0 g Fiber;

Salmon Cucumber Rolls

Preparation Time: 15 minutes;

Cooking Time: 0 minutes;

Servings: 2

Ingredients

- 1 large cucumber
- 2 oz. smoked salmon
- 4 tbsp. mayonnaise
- 1 tsp sesame seeds
- Seasoning:
- ¼ tsp salt
- ¼ tsp ground black pepper

Directions:

1. Trim the ends of the cucumber, cut it into slices by using a vegetable peeler, and then place half of the cucumber slices in a dish.
2. Cover with paper towels, layer with remaining cucumber slices, top with paper towels, and let them refrigerate for 5 minutes.
3. Meanwhile, take a medium bowl, place salmon in it, add mayonnaise, season with salt and black pepper, and then stir until well combined.
4. Remove cucumber slices from the refrigerator, place salmon on one side of each cucumber slice, and then roll tightly.
5. Repeat with remaining cucumber, sprinkle with sesame seeds and then serve.

Nutrition: 269 Calories; 24 g Fats; 6.7 g Protein; 4 g Net Carb; 2 g Fiber;

Bacon Wrapped Mahi-Mahi

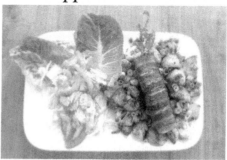

Preparation Time: 10 minutes

Cooking Time: 12 minutes;

Servings: 2

Ingredients

2 fillets of mahi-mahi

2 strips of bacon

½ of lime, zested

4 basil leaves

½ tsp salt

Seasoning:

½ tsp ground black pepper

1 tbsp. avocado oil

Directions:

1. Turn on the oven, then set it to 375 degrees F and let them preheat.
2. Meanwhile, season fillets with salt and black pepper, top each fillet with 2 basil leaves, sprinkle with lime zest, wrap with a bacon strip and secure with a toothpick if needed.
3. Take a medium skillet pan, place it over medium-high heat, add oil and when hot, place prepared fillets in it and cook for 2 minutes per side.
4. Transfer pan into the oven and bake the fish for 5 to 7 minutes until thoroughly cooked.
5. Serve.

Nutrition: 217 Calories; 11.3 g Fats; 27.1 g Protein; 1.2 g Net Carb; 0.5 g Fiber;

Cheesy Garlic Bread with Smoked Salmon

Preparation Time: 10 minutes

Cooking Time: 1 minute;

Servings: 2

Ingredients

- 4 tbsp. almond flour
- ½ tsp baking powder
- 2 tbsp. grated cheddar cheese
- 1 egg
- 2 oz. salmon, cut into thin sliced
- Seasoning:
- 1 tbsp. butter, unsalted
- ¼ tsp garlic powder
- 1/8 tsp salt
- ¼ tsp Italian seasoning

Directions:

1. Take a heatproof bowl, place all the ingredients in it except for cheese and then stir by using a fork until well combined.
2. Fold in cheese until just mixed and then microwave for 1 minute at high heat setting until thoroughly cooked, else continue cooking for another 15 to 30 seconds.
3. When done, lift out the bread, cool it for 5 minutes and then cut it into slices.
4. Top each slice with salmon and then serve straight away

Nutrition: 233 Calories; 18 g Fats; 13.8 g Protein; 1.9 g Net Carb; 1.5 g Fiber;

Smoked Salmon Pasta Salad

Preparation Time: 10 minutes

Cooking Time: 0 minutes;

Servings: 2

Ingredients

- 1 zucchini, spiralized into noodles
- 4 oz. smoked salmon, break into pieces
- 2 oz. cream cheese
- 2 oz. mayonnaise
- 2 oz. sour cream
- Seasoning:
- 1/3 tsp salt
- ¼ tsp ground black pepper
- ¼ tsp hot sauce

Directions:

1. Take a medium bowl, place cream cheese in it, add mayonnaise, sour cream, salt, black pepper and hot sauce and stir until well combined.
2. Add zucchini noodles, toss until well coated and then fold in salmon until just mixed.
3. Serve.

Nutrition: 458 Calories; 38.7 g Fats; 15.4 g Protein; 6.1 g Net Carb; 1.7 g Fiber;

Tuna Salad Pickle Boats

Preparation Time: 10 minutes

Cooking Time: 0 minutes;

Servings: 2

Ingredients

- 4 dill pickles
- 4 oz. of tuna, packed in water, drained
- ¼ of lime, juiced
- 4 tbsp. mayonnaise
- Seasoning:
- ¼ tsp salt
- 1/8 tsp ground black pepper
- ¼ tsp paprika
- 1 tbsp. mustard paste

Directions:

1. Prepare tuna salad and for this, take a medium bowl, place tuna in it, add lime juice, mayonnaise, salt, black pepper, paprika, and mustard and stir until mixed.
2. Cut each pickle into half lengthwise, scoop out seeds, and then fill with tuna salad.
3. Serve.

Nutrition: 308.5 Calories; 23.7 g Fats; 17 g Protein; 3.8 g Net Carb; 3.1 g Fiber;

Shrimp Deviled Eggs

Preparation Time: 5 minutes
Cooking Time: 0 minutes;
Servings: 2
Ingredients

- 2 eggs, boiled
- 2 oz. shrimps, cooked, chopped
- ½ tsp tabasco sauce
- ½ tsp mustard paste
- 2 tbsp. mayonnaise
- Seasoning:
- 1/8 tsp salt
- 1/8 tsp ground black pepper

Directions:

1. Peel the boiled eggs, then slice in half lengthwise and transfer egg yolks to a medium bowl by using a spoon.
2. Mash the egg yolk, add remaining ingredients and stir until well combined.
3. Spoon the egg yolk mixture into egg whites, and then serve.

Nutrition: 210 Calories; 16.4 g Fats; 14 g Protein; 1 g Net Carb; 0.1 g Fiber;

Herb Crusted Tilapia

Preparation Time: 5 minutes
Cooking Time: 10 minutes;
Servings: 2
Ingredients

- 2 fillets of tilapia
- ½ tsp garlic powder
- ½ tsp Italian seasoning
- ½ tsp dried parsley
- 1/3 tsp salt
- Seasoning:
- 2 tbsp. melted butter, unsalted
- 1 tbsp. avocado oil

Directions:

1. Turn on the broiler and then let it preheat.
2. Meanwhile, take a small bowl, place melted butter in it, stir in oil and garlic powder until mixed, and then brush this mixture over tilapia fillets.
3. Stir together remaining spices and then sprinkle them generously on tilapia until well coated.
4. Place seasoned tilapia in a baking pan, place the pan under the broiler and then bake for 10 minutes until tender and golden, brushing with garlic-butter every 2 minutes.
5. Serve.

Nutrition: 520 Calories; 35 g Fats; 36.2 g Protein; 13.6 g Net Carb; 0.6 g Fiber;

Tuna Stuffed Avocado

Preparation Time: 5 minutes
Cooking Time: 0 minutes;
Servings: 2
Ingredients

- 1 medium avocado

- ¼ of a lemon, juiced
- 5-ounce tuna, packed in water
- 1 green onion, chopped
- 2 slices of turkey bacon, cooked, crumbled
- Seasoning:
- ¼ tsp salt
- ¼ tsp ground black pepper

Directions:

1. Drain tuna, place it in a bowl, and then broke it into pieces with a form.
2. Add remaining ingredients, except for avocado and bacon, and stir until well combined.
3. Cut avocado into half, remove its pit and then stuff its cavity evenly with the tuna mixture.
4. Top stuffed avocados with bacon and Serve.

Nutrition: 108.5 Calories; 8 g Fats; 6 g Protein; 0.8 g Net Carb; 2.3 g Fiber;

Garlic Butter Salmon

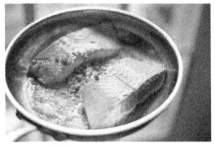

Preparation Time: 10 minutes
Cooking Time: 15 minutes
Servings: 2
Ingredients

- 2 salmon fillets, skinless
- 1 tsp minced garlic
- 1 tbsp. chopped cilantro
- 1 tbsp. unsalted butter
- 2 tbsp. grated cheddar cheese
- Seasoning:
- ½ tsp salt
- ¼ tsp ground black pepper

Directions:

1. Turn on the oven, then set it to 350 degrees F, and let it preheat.
2. Meanwhile, taking a rimmed baking sheet, grease it with oil, place salmon fillets on it, season with salt and black pepper on both sides.
3. Stir together butter, cilantro, and cheese until combined, then coat the mixture on both sides of salmon in an even layer and bake for 15 minutes until thoroughly cooked.
4. Then Turn on the broiler and continue baking the salmon for 2 minutes until the top is golden brown.
5. Serve.

Nutrition: 128 Calories; 4.5 g Fats; 41 g Protein; 1 g Net Carb; 0 g Fiber;

CHAPTER 10:

Vegetables

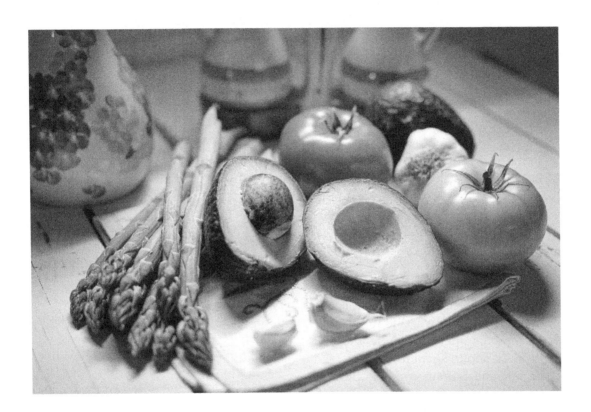

Portobello Mushroom Pizza

Preparation Time: 15 minutes

Cooking Time: 5 minutes

Servings: 4

Ingredients:

- 4 large portobello mushrooms, stems removed
- ¼ cup olive oil
- 1 teaspoon minced garlic
- 1 medium tomato, cut into 4 slices
- 2 teaspoons chopped fresh basil
- 1 cup shredded mozzarella cheese

Directions:

1. Preheat the oven to broil. Line a baking sheet with aluminum foil and set aside.
2. In a small bowl, toss the mushroom caps with the olive oil until well coated. Use your fingertips to rub the oil in without breaking the mushrooms.
3. Place the mushrooms on the baking sheet gill-side down and broil the mushrooms until they are tender on the tops, about 2 minute
4. Flip the mushrooms over and broil 1 minute more
5. Take the baking sheet out and spread the garlic over each mushroom, top each with a tomato slice, sprinkle with the basil, and top with the cheese
6. Broil the mushrooms until the cheese is melted and bubbly, about 1 minute.
7. Serve.

Nutrition:

Calories: 251

Fat: 20g

Protein: 14g

Carbs: 7g

Fiber: 3g Net Carbs: 4g

Fat 71 Protein 19

Carbs 10

Garlicky Green Beans

Preparation Time: 10 minutes

Cooking Time: 10 minutes

Servings: 4

Ingredients:

- 1 pound green beans, stemmed
- 2 tablespoons olive oil
- 1 teaspoon minced garlic
- Sea salt
- Freshly ground black pepper
- ¼ cup freshly grated Parmesan cheese

Directions:

1. Preheat the oven to 425°F. Line a baking sheet with aluminum foil and set aside.
2. In a large bowl, toss together the green beans, olive oil, and garlic until well mixed.
3. Season the beans lightly with salt and pepper
4. Spread the beans on the baking sheet and roast them until they are tender and lightly browned, stirring them once, about 10 minutes.
5. Serve topped with the Parmesan cheese.

Nutrition:

Calories: 104 Fat: 9g

Protein: 4g Carbs: 2g

Fiber: 1g Net Carbs: 1g

Fat 77 Protein 15

Carbs 8

Sautéed Asparagus with Walnuts

Preparation Time: 10 minutes

Cooking Time: 5 minutes

Servings: 4

Ingredients:

- 1½ tablespoons olive oil
- ¾ pound asparagus, woody ends trimmed
- Sea salt
- Freshly ground pepper
- ¼ cup chopped walnuts

Directions:

1. Place a large skillet over medium-high heat and add the olive oil.
2. Sauté the asparagus until the spears are tender and lightly browned, about 5 minutes.
3. Season the asparagus with salt and pepper.
4. Remove the skillet from the heat and toss the asparagus with the walnuts.
5. Serve.

Nutrition:

Calories: 124 Fat: 12g

Protein: 3g Carbs: 4g

Fiber: 2g

Net Carbs: 2g

Fat 81

Protein

Carbs 10

Brussels Sprouts Casserole

Preparation Time: 15 minutes

Cooking Time: 30 minutes

Servings: 8

Ingredients:

- 8 bacon slices
- 1 pound Brussels sprouts, blanched for 10 minutes and cut into quarters
- 1 cup shredded Swiss cheese, divided
- ¾ cup heavy (whipping) cream

Directions:

1. Preheat the oven to 400°F.
2. Place a skillet over medium-high heat and cook the bacon until it is crispy, about 6 minutes.
3. Reserve 1 tablespoon of bacon fat to grease the casserole dish and roughly chop the cooked bacon.
4. Lightly oil a casserole dish with the reserved bacon fat and set aside.
5. In a medium bowl, toss the Brussels sprouts with the chopped bacon and ½ cup of cheese and transfer the mixture to the casserole dish.
6. Pour the heavy cream over the Brussels sprouts and top the casserole with the remaining ½ cup of cheese.
7. Bake until the cheese is melted and lightly browned and the vegetables are heated through, about 20 minutes.
8. Serve.

Nutrition:

Calories: 299

Fat: 11g

Protein: 12g

Carbs: 7g

Fiber: 3g

Net Carbs: 4g

Fat 77

Protein 15

Carbs 8

Creamed Spinach

Preparation Time: 10 minutes

Cooking Time: 30 minutes

Servings: 4

Ingredients:

- 1 tablespoon butter
- ½ sweet onion, very thinly sliced
- 4 cups spinach, stemmed and thoroughly washed
- ¾ cup heavy (whipping) cream
- ¼ cup Herbed Chicken Stock (here)
- Pinch sea salt
- Pinch freshly ground black pepper
- Pinch ground nutmeg

Directions:

1. In a large skillet over medium heat, add the butter.
2. Sauté the onion until it is lightly caramelized, about 5 minutes.
3. Stir in the spinach, heavy cream, chicken stock, salt, pepper, and nutmeg.
4. Sauté until the spinach is wilted, about 5 minutes.
5. Continue cooking the spinach until it is tender and the sauce is thickened, about 15 minutes.
6. Serve immediately.

Nutrition:

Calories: 195

Fat: 20g

Protein: 3g

Carbs: 3g

Fiber: 2g

Net Carbs: 1g

Fat 88

Protein 6

Carbs 6

Cheesy Mashed Cauliflower

Preparation Time: 15 minutes

Cooking Time: 5 minutes

Servings: 4

Ingredients:

- 1 head cauliflower, chopped roughly
- ½ cup shredded Cheddar cheese
- ¼ cup heavy (whipping) cream
- 2 tablespoons butter, at room temperature
- Sea salt
- Freshly ground black pepper

Directions:

1. Place a large saucepan filled three-quarters full with water over high heat and bring to a boil.
2. Blanch the cauliflower until tender, about 5 minutes, and drain.
3. Transfer the cauliflower to a food processor and add the cheese, heavy cream, and butter. Purée until very creamy and whipped.
4. Season with salt and pepper.
5. Serve.

Nutrition:

Calories: 183

Fat: 15g

Protein: 8g

Carbs: 6g

Fiber: 2g

Net Carbs: 4g

Fat 75

Protein 14

Carbs 11

Sautéed Crispy Zucchini

Preparation Time: 15 minutes

Cooking Time: 10 minutes

Servings: 4

Ingredients:

- 2 tablespoons butter
- 4 zucchini, cut into ¼-inch-thick rounds
- ½ cup freshly grated Parmesan cheese
- Freshly ground black pepper

Directions:

1. Place a large skillet over medium-high heat and melt the butter.
2. Add the zucchini and sauté until tender and lightly browned, about 5 minutes.
3. Spread the zucchini evenly in the skillet and sprinkle the Parmesan cheese over the vegetables.
4. Cook without stirring until the Parmesan cheese is melted and crispy where it touches the skillet, about 5 minutes.
5. Serve.

Nutrition:

Calories: 94

Fat: 8g

Protein: 4g

Carbs: 1g

Fiber: 0g

Net Carbs: 1g

Fat 76

Protein 20

Carbs 4

Mushrooms with Camembert

Preparation Time: 5 minutes

Cooking Time: 15 minutes

Servings: 4

Ingredients:

- 2 tablespoons butter
- 2 teaspoons minced garlic
- 1 pound button mushrooms, halved
- 4 ounces Camembert cheese, diced
- Freshly ground black pepper

Directions:

1. Place a large skillet over medium-high heat and melt the butter.
2. Sauté the garlic until translucent, about 3 minutes.
3. Sauté the mushrooms until tender, about 10 minutes.
4. Stir in the cheese and sauté until melted, about 2 minutes.
5. Season with pepper and serve.

Nutrition:

Calories: 161

Fat: 13g

Protein: 9g

Carbs: 4g

Fiber: 1g

Net Carbs: 3g

Fat 70

Protein 21

Carbs 9

Pesto Zucchini Noodles

Preparation Time: 15 minutes

Cooking Time: 10 minutes

Servings: 4

Ingredients:

- 4 small zucchini, ends trimmed

- ¾ cup Herb Kale Pesto (here) ¼ cup grated or shredded
- Parmesan chees

Directions:

1. Use a spiralizer or peeler to cut the zucchini into "noodles" and place them in a medium bowl.
2. Add the pesto and the Parmesan cheese and toss to coat.
3. Serve.

Nutrition:

Calories: 93
Fat: 8g
Protein: 4g
Carbs: 2g
Fiber: 0g
Net Carbs: 2g
Fat 70
Protein 15
Carbs 8

Golden Rosti

Preparation Time: 15 minutes
Cooking Time: 15 minutes
Servings: 8
Ingredients:

- 8 bacon slices, chopped
- 1 cup shredded acorn squash
- 1 cup shredded raw celeriac
- 2 tablespoons grated or shredded Parmesan cheese
- 2 teaspoons minced garlic
- 1 teaspoon chopped fresh thyme
- Sea salt
- Freshly ground black pepper
- 2 tablespoons butter

Directions:

1. In a large skillet over medium-high heat, cook the bacon until crispy, about 5 minutes.
2. While the bacon is cooking, in a large bowl, mix together the squash, celeriac, Parmesan cheese, garlic, and thyme. Season the mixture generously with salt and pepper, and set aside.
3. Remove the cooked bacon with a slotted spoon to the rosti mixture and stir to incorporate.
4. Remove all but 2 tablespoons of bacon fat from the skillet and add the butter
5. Reduce the heat to medium-low and transfer the rosti mixture to the skillet and spread it out evenly to form a large round patty about 1 inch thick.
6. Cook until the bottom of the rosti is golden brown and crisp, about 5 minutes.
7. Flip the rosti over and cook until the other side is crispy and the middle is cooked through, about 5 minutes more.
8. Remove the skillet from the heat and cut the rosti into 8 pieces
9. Serve.

Nutrition:

Calories: 171
Fat: 15g
Protein: 5g
Carbs: 3g
Fiber: 0g
Net Carbs: 3g
Fat 81
Protein 12
Carbs 7

Artichoke and Avocado Pasta Salad

Preparation Time: 15 minutes

Cooking Time: 30 minutes

Servings: 10 servings

Ingredients:

- Two cups of spiral pasta (uncooked)
- A quarter cup of Romano cheese (grated)
- One can (fourteen oz.) of artichoke hearts (coarsely chopped and drained well)
- One avocado (medium-sized, ripe, cubed)
- Two plum tomatoes (chopped coarsely)

For the dressing:

- One tbsp. of fresh cilantro (chopped)
- Two tbsps. of lime juice
- A quarter cup of canola oil
- One and a half tsps. of lime zest (grated)
- Half a tsp. each of
- Pepper (freshly ground)
- Kosher salt

Directions:

1. Follow the directions mentioned on the package for cooking the pasta. Drain them well and rinse using cold water.
2. Then, take a large-sized bowl and in it, add the pasta along with the tomatoes, artichoke hearts, cheese, and avocado. Combine them well. Then, take another bowl and add all the ingredients of the dressing in it. Whisk them together and, once combined, add the dressing over the pasta.
3. Gently toss the mixture to coat everything evenly in the dressing and then refrigerate.

Nutrition:

Calories: 188

Protein: 6g

Fat: 10g

Carbs: 21g

Fiber: 2g

Apple Arugula and Turkey Salad in a Jar

Preparation Time: 10 minutes

Cooking Time: 10 minutes

Servings: 4 servings

Ingredients:

- Three tbsps. of red wine vinegar
- Two tbsps. of chives (freshly minced)
- Half a cup of orange juice
- One to three tbsps. of sesame oil
- A quarter tsp. each of
- Pepper (coarsely ground)
- Salt

For the salad:

- Four tsps. of curry powder
- Four cups each of
- Turkey (cubed, cooked)
- Baby spinach or fresh arugula
- A quarter tsp. of salt
- Half a tsp. of pepper (coarsely ground)
- One cup of halved green grapes
- One apple (large-sized, chopped)
- Eleven oz. of mandarin oranges (properly drained)
- One tbsp. of lemon juice
- Half a cup each of

- Walnuts (chopped)
- Dried cranberries or pomegranate seeds

Directions:

1. Take a small-sized bowl and, in it, add the first 6 ingredients from the list into it. Whisk them. Then take a large bowl and in it, add the turkey and then add the seasonings on top of it. Toss the turkey cubes to coat them with the seasoning. Take another bowl and in it, add the lemon juice and toss the apple chunks in the juice.

2. Take four jars and divide the layers in the order I mention here - first goes the orange juice mixture, the second layer is that of the turkey, then apple, oranges, grapes, cranberries or pomegranate seeds, walnuts, and spinach or arugula. Cover the jars and then refrigerate them.

Nutrition:

Calories: 471

Protein: 45g

Fat: 19g

Carbs: 33g

Fiber: 5g

CHAPTER 11:

Snacks

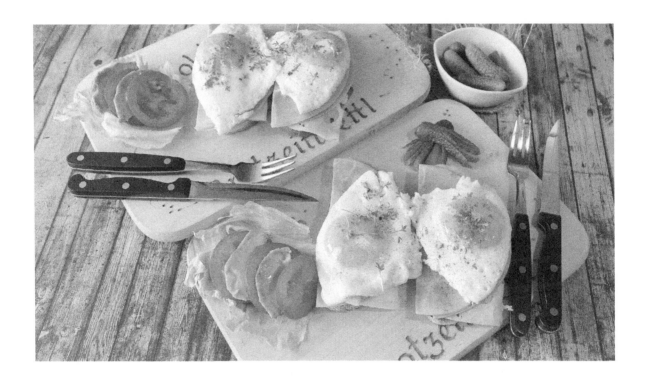

Fluffy Bites

Preparation Time: 20 minutes

Cooking Time: 60 minutes

Servings: 12

Ingredients:

- 2 Teaspoons Cinnamon
- 2/3 Cup Sour Cream
- 2 Cups Heavy Cream
- 1 Teaspoon Scraped Vanilla Bean
- ¼ Teaspoon Cardamom
- 4 Egg Yolks
- Stevia to Taste

Directions:

1. Start by whisking your egg yolks until creamy and smooth.
2. Get out a double boiler, and add your eggs with the rest of your ingredients. Mix well.
3. Remove from heat, allowing it to cool until it reaches room temperature.
4. Refrigerate for an hour before whisking well.
5. Pour into molds, and freeze for at least an hour before serving.

Nutrition:

Calories: 363

Protein: 2

Fat: 40

Carbohydrates: 1

Coconut Fudge

Preparation Time: 20 minutes

Cooking Time: 60 minutes

Servings: 12

Ingredients:

- 2 Cups Coconut Oil
- ½ Cup Dark Cocoa Powder
- ½ Cup Coconut Cream
- ¼ Cup Almonds, Chopped
- ¼ Cup Coconut, Shredded
- 1 Teaspoon Almond Extract
- Pinch of Salt
- Stevia to Taste

Directions:

1. Pour your coconut oil and coconut cream in a bowl, whisking with an electric beater until smooth. Once the mixture becomes smooth and glossy, do not continue.
2. Begin to add in your cocoa powder while mixing slowly, making sure that there aren't any lumps.
3. Add in the rest of your ingredients, and mix well.
4. Line a bread pan with parchment paper, and freeze until it sets.
5. Slice into squares before serving.

Nutrition:

Calories: 172

Fat: 20

Carbohydrates: 3

Nutmeg Nougat

Preparation Time: 30 minutes

Cooking Time: 60 minutes

Servings: 12

Ingredients:

- 1 Cup Heavy Cream
- 1 Cup Cashew Butter
- 1 Cup Coconut, Shredded
- ½ Teaspoon Nutmeg
- 1 Teaspoon Vanilla Extract, Pure
- Stevia to Taste

Directions:

1. Melt your cashew butter using a double boiler, and then stir in your vanilla extract, dairy cream, nutmeg and stevia. Make sure it's mixed well.
2. Remove from heat, allowing it to cooldown before refrigerating it for a half hour.
3. Shape into balls, and coat with shredded coconut. Chill for at least two hours before serving.

Nutrition:

Calories: 341

Fat: 34

Carbohydrates: 5

Sweet Almond Bites

Preparation Time: 30 minutes

Cooking Time: 90 minutes

Servings: 12

Ingredients:

- 18 Ounces Butter, Grass Fed
- 2 Ounces Heavy Cream
- ½ Cup Stevia
- 2/3 Cup Cocoa Powder
- 1 Teaspoon Vanilla Extract, Pure
- 4 Tablespoons Almond Butter

Direction:

1. Use a double boiler to melt your butter before adding in all of your remaining ingredients.
2. Place the mixture into molds, freezing for two hours before serving.

Nutrition:

Calories: 350

Protein: 2

Fat: 38

Strawberry Cheesecake Minis

Preparation Time: 30 minutes

Cooking Time: 120 minutes

Servings: 12

Ingredients:

- 1 Cup Coconut Oil
- 1 Cup Coconut Butter
- ½ Cup Strawberries, Sliced
- ½ Teaspoon Lime Juice
- 2 Tablespoons Cream Cheese, Full Fat
- Stevia to Taste

Directions:

1. Blend your strawberries together.
2. Soften your cream cheese, and then add in your coconut butter.
3. Combine all ingredients together, and then pour your mixture into silicone molds.
4. Freeze for at least two hours before serving.

Nutrition:

Calories: 372 Protein: 1

Fat: 41 Carbohydrates: 2

Cocoa Brownies

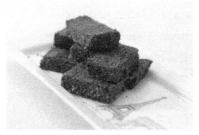

Preparation Time: 10 minutes

Cooking Time: 30 minutes

Servings: 12

Ingredients:

- 1 Egg

- 2 Tablespoons Butter, Grass Fed
- 2 Teaspoons Vanilla Extract, Pure
- ¼ Teaspoon Baking Powder
- ¼ Cup Cocoa Powder
- 1/3 Cup Heavy Cream
- ¾ Cup Almond Butter
- Pinch Sea Salt

Directions:

1. Break your egg into a bowl, whisking until smooth.
2. Add in all of your wet ingredients, mixing well.
3. Mix all dry ingredients into a bowl.
4. Sift your dry ingredients into your wet ingredients, mixing to form a batter.
5. Get out a baking pan, greasing it before pouring in your mixture.
6. Heat your oven to 350 and bake for twenty-five minutes.
7. Allow it to cool before slicing and serve room temperature or warm.

Nutrition:

Calories: 184

Protein: 1

Fat: 20

Carbohydrates: 1

Chocolate Orange Bites

Preparation Time: 20 minutes

Cooking Time: 120 minutes

Servings: 6

Ingredients:

- 10 Ounces Coconut Oil
- 4 Tablespoons Cocoa Powder
- ¼ Teaspoon Blood Orange Extract
- Stevia to Taste

Directions:

1. Melt half of your coconut oil using a double boiler, and then add in your stevia and orange extract.
2. Get out candy molds, pouring the mixture into it. Fill each mold halfway, and then place in the fridge until they set.
3. Melt the other half of your coconut oil, stirring in your cocoa powder and stevia, making sure that the mixture is smooth with no lumps.
4. Pour into your molds, filling them up all the way, and then allow it to set in the fridge before serving.

Nutrition:

Calories: *188*

Protein: *1*

Fat: 21

Carbohydrates: 5

Caramel Cones

Preparation Time: 25 minutes

Cooking Time: 120 minutes

Servings: 6

Ingredients:

- 2 Tablespoons Heavy Whipping Cream
- 2 Tablespoons Sour Cream
- 1 Tablespoon Caramel Sugar
- 1 Teaspoon Sea Salt, Fine
- 1/3 Cup Butter, Grass Fed
- 1/3 Cup Coconut Oil
- Stevia to Taste

Directions:

1. Soften your coconut oil and butter, mixing together.

2. Mix all ingredients together to form a batter, and ten place them in molds.
3. Top with a little salt, and keep refrigerated until serving.

Nutrition:

Calories: *100* Fat: 12 Grams

Carbohydrates: 1

Cinnamon Bites

Preparation Time: 20 minutes

Cooking Time: 95 minutes

Servings: 6

Ingredients:

- 1/8 Teaspoon Nutmeg
- 1 Teaspoon Vanilla Extract
- ¼ Teaspoon Cinnamon
- 4 Tablespoons Coconut Oil
- ½ Cup Butter, Grass Fed
- 8 Ounces Cream Cheese
- Stevia to Taste

Directions:

1. Soften your coconut oil and butter, mixing in your cream cheese.
2. Add all of your remaining ingredients, and mix well.
3. Pour into molds, and freeze until set.

Nutrition:

Calories: *178* Protein: *1*

Fat: 19

Sweet Chai Bites

Preparation Time: 20 minutes

Cooking Time: 45 minutes

Servings: 6

Ingredients:

- 1 Cup Cream Cheese
- 1 Cup Coconut Oil
- 2 Ounces Butter, Grass Fed
- 2 Teaspoons Ginger
- 2 Teaspoons Cardamom
- 1 Teaspoon Nutmeg
- 1 Teaspoon Cloves
- 1 Teaspoon Vanilla Extract, Pure
- 1 Teaspoon Darjeeling Black Tea
- Stevia to Taste

Directions:

1. Melt your coconut oil and butter before adding in your black tea. Allow it to set for one to two minutes.
2. Add in your cream cheese, removing your mixture from heat.
3. Add in all of your spices, and stir to combine.
4. Pour into molds, and freeze before serving.

Nutrition:

Calories: *178*

Protein: *1*

Fat: 19

Easy Vanilla Bombs

Preparation Time: 20 minutes

Cooking Time: 45 minutes

Servings: 14

Ingredients:

- 1 Cup Macadamia Nuts, Unsalted
- ¼ Cup Coconut Oil / ¼ Cup Butter
- 2 Teaspoons Vanilla Extract, Sugar Free
- 20 Drops Liquid Stevia
- 2 Tablespoons Erythritol, Powdered

Directions:

1. Pulse your macadamia nuts in a blender, and then combine all of your ingredients together. Mix well.
2. Get out mini muffin tins with a tablespoon and a half of the mixture.
3. Refrigerate it for a half hour before serving.

Nutrition:

Calories: 125

Fat: 5

Carbohydrates: 5

Marinated Eggs.

Preparation Time: 2 hours and 10 minutes

Cooking Time: 7 minutes

Servings: 4

Ingredients:

- 6 eggs
- 1 and ¼ cups water
- ¼ cup unsweetened rice vinegar 2 tablespoons coconut aminos
- Salt and black pepper to the taste 2 garlic cloves, minced
- 1 teaspoon stevia 4 ounces cream cheese
- 1 tablespoon chives, chopped

Directions:

1. Put the eggs in a pot, add water to cover, bring to a boil over medium heat, cover and cook for 7 minutes.
2. Rinse eggs with cold water and leave them aside to cool down.
3. In a bowl, mix 1 cup water with coconut aminos, vinegar, stevia and garlic and whisk well.
4. Put the eggs in this mix, cover with a kitchen towel and leave them aside for 2 hours rotating from time to time.

5. Peel eggs, cut in halves and put egg yolks in a bowl.
6. Add ¼ cup water, cream cheese, salt, pepper and chives and stir well.
7. Stuff egg whites with this mix and serve them.
8. Enjoy!

Nutrition:

Calories: 289 kcal

Protein: 15.86 g

Fat: 22.62 g

Carbohydrates: 4.52 g

Sodium: 288 mg

Sausage and Cheese Dip.

Preparation Time: 10 minutes

Cooking Time: 130 minutes

Servings: 28

Ingredients:

- 8 ounces cream cheese
- A pinch of salt and black pepper
- 16 ounces sour cream
- 8 ounces pepper jack cheese, chopped
- 15 ounces canned tomatoes mixed with habaneros
- 1 pound Italian sausage, ground
- ¼ cup green onions, chopped

Directions:

1. Heat up a pan over medium heat, add sausage, stir and cook until it browns.
2. Add tomatoes mix, stir and cook for 4 minutes more.
3. Add a pinch of salt, pepper and the green onions, stir and cook for 4 minutes.
4. Spread pepper jack cheese on the bottom of your slow cooker.

5. Add cream cheese, sausage mix and sour cream, cover and cook on High for 2 hours.
6. Uncover your slow cooker, stir dip, transfer to a bowl and serve.
7. Enjoy!

Nutrition:

Calories: 132 kcal

Protein: 6.79 g

Fat: 9.58 g

Carbohydrates: 6.22 g

Sodium: 362 mg

Tasty Onion and Cauliflower Dip.

Preparation Time: 20 minutes

Cooking Time: 30 minutes

Servings: 24

Ingredients:

- 1 and ½ cups chicken stock
- 1 cauliflower head, florets separated
- ¼ cup mayonnaise
- ½ cup yellow onion, chopped
- ¾ cup cream cheese
- ½ teaspoon chili powder
- ½ teaspoon cumin, ground
- ½ teaspoon garlic powder
- Salt and black pepper to the taste

Directions:

1. Put the stock in a pot, add cauliflower and onion, heat up over medium heat and cook for 30 minutes.
2. Add chili powder, salt, pepper, cumin and garlic powder and stir.
3. Also add cream cheese and stir a bit until it melts.
4. Blend using an immersion blender and mix with the mayo.

5. Transfer to a bowl and keep in the fridge for 2 hours before you serve it.
6. Enjoy!

Nutrition:

Calories: 40 kcal Protein: 1.23 g

Fat: 3.31 g Carbohydrates: 1.66 g

Sodium: 72 mg

Pesto Crackers.

Preparation Time: 10 minutes

Cooking Time: 17 minutes

Servings: 6

Ingredients

- ½ teaspoon baking powder
- Salt and black pepper to the taste
- 1 and ¼ cups almond flour ¼ teaspoon basil, dried 1 garlic clove, minced
- 2 tablespoons basil pesto
- A pinch of cayenne pepper
- 3 tablespoons ghee

Directions:

1. In a bowl, mix salt, pepper, baking powder and almond flour.
2. Add garlic, cayenne and basil and stir.
3. Add pesto and whisk.
4. Also add ghee and mix your dough with your finger.
5. Spread this dough on a lined baking sheet, introduce in the oven at 325 degrees F and bake for 17 minutes.
6. Leave aside to cool down, cut your crackers and serve them as a snack.
7. Enjoy!

Nutrition:

Calories: 9 kcal Protein: 0.41 g

Fat: 0.14 g Carbohydrates: 1.86 g

Sodium: 2 mg

Pumpkin Muffins.

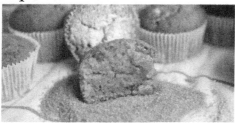

Preparation Time: 10 minutes

Cooking Time: 15 minutes

Servings: 18

Ingredients:

- ¼ cup sunflower seed butter
- ¾ cup pumpkin puree 2 tablespoons flaxseed meal ¼ cup coconut flour
- ½ cup erythritol ½ teaspoon nutmeg, ground
- 1 teaspoon cinnamon, ground ½ teaspoon baking soda 1 egg ½ teaspoon baking powder
- A pinch of salt

Directions:

1. In a bowl, mix butter with pumpkin puree and egg and blend well.
2. Add flaxseed meal, coconut flour, erythritol, baking soda, baking powder, nutmeg, cinnamon and a pinch of salt and stir well.
3. Spoon this into a greased muffin pan, introduce in the oven at 350 degrees F and bake for 15 minutes.
4. Leave muffins to cool down and serve them as a snack.
5. Enjoy!

Nutrition:

Calories: 65 kcal

Protein: 2.82 g

Fat: 5.42 g

Carbohydrates: 2.27 g

Sodium: 57 mg

Creamy Mango and Mint Dip

Preparation Time: 10 minutes

Cooking Time: 15 minutes

Servings 4

Ingredients:

- Medium green chili, chopped – 1
- Medium white onion, peeled and chopped – 1
- Grated ginger – 1 tablespoon
- Minced garlic – 1 teaspoon
- Salt – 1/8 teaspoon
- Ground black pepper – 1/8 teaspoon
- Cumin powder – 1 teaspoon
- Mango powder – 1 teaspoon
- Mint leaves – 2 cups
- Coriander leaves – 1 cup
- Cashew yogurt – 4 tablespoons

Directions:

1. Place all the ingredients for the dip in a blender and pulse for 1 to 2 minutes or until smooth.
2. Tip the dip into small cups and serve straightaway.

Nutrition: calories: 100, fat: 2, fiber: 3, carbs: 7, protein: 5

Hot Red Chili and Garlic Chutney

Preparation Time: 25 minutes

Cooking Time: 15 minutes

Servings 1

Ingredients:

- Red chilies, dried – 14
- Minced garlic – 5 teaspoons
- Salt – 1/8 teaspoon
- Water – 1 and ¼ cups

Directions:

1. Place chilies in a bowl, pour in water and let rest for 20 minutes.
2. Then drain red chilies, chop them and add to a blender. Add remaining ingredients into the blender and pulse for 1 to 2 minutes until smooth. Tip the sauce into a bowl and serve straight away.

Nutrition: calories: 100, fat: 1, fiber: 2, carbs: 6, protein: 7

Red Chilies and Onion Chutney

Preparation Time: 15 minutes

Cooking Time: 15 minutes

Servings 2

Ingredients:

- Medium white onion, peeled and chopped – 1
- Minced garlic – 1 teaspoon
- Red chilies, chopped – 2
- Salt – ¼ teaspoon
- Sweet paprika – 1 teaspoon
- Avocado oil – 2 teaspoons
- Water – ¼ cup

Directions:

1. Place a medium skillet pan over medium-high heat, add oil and when hot, add onion, garlic, and chilies.
2. Cook onions for 5 minutes or until softened, then season with salt and paprika and pour in water. Stir well and cook for 5 minutes. Then spoon the chutney into a bowl and serve.

Nutrition: calories: 121, fat: 2, fiber: 6, carbs: 9, protein: 5

Fast Guacamole

Preparation Time: 10 minutes

Cooking Time: 15 minutes

Servings 12

Ingredients:

- Medium avocados, peeled, pitted and cubed – 3
- Medium tomato, cubed – 1
- Chopped cilantro – ¼ cup
- Medium red onion, peeled and chopped – 1
- Salt – ½ teaspoon
- Ground white pepper – ¼ teaspoon
- Lime juice – 3 tablespoons

Directions:

1. Place all the ingredients for the salad in a medium bowl and stir until combined.
2. Serve guacamole straightaway as an appetizer.

Nutrition: calories: 87, fat: 4, fiber: 4, carbs: 8, protein: 2

Coconut Dill Dip

Preparation Time: 10 minutes

Cooking Time: 15 minutes

Servings 10

Ingredients:

- Chopped white onion – 1 tablespoon
- Parsley flakes – 2 teaspoons
- Chopped dill – 2 teaspoons
- Salt – ¼ teaspoon
- Coconut cream – 1 cup
- Avocado mayonnaise – ½ cup

Directions:

1. Place all the ingredients for the dip in a medium bowl and whisk until combined.Serve the dip with vegetable sticks as a side dish.

Nutrition: calories: 102, fat: 3, fiber: 1, carbs: 2, protein: 2

Creamy Crab Dip

Preparation Time 5 minutes

Cooking Time: 10 minutes

Servings 12

Ingredients:

- Crab meat, chopped – 1 pound
- Chopped white onion – 2 tablespoons
- Minced garlic – 1 tablespoon
- Lemon juice – 2 tablespoons
- Cream cheese, cubed – 16 ounces
- Avocado mayonnaise – 1/3 cup
- Grape juice – 2 tablespoons

Directions:

1. Place all the ingredients for the dip in a medium bowl and stir until combined.
2. Divide dip evenly between small bowls and serve as a party dip.

Nutrition: Calories: 100, Fat: 4, Fiber: 1, Carbs: 4, Protein: 4

Creamy Cheddar and Bacon Spread with Almonds

Preparation Time: 10 minutes

Cooking Time: 10 minutes

Servings 12

Ingredients:

- Bacon, cooked and chopped – 12 ounces

- Chopped sweet red pepper – 2 tablespoons
- Medium white onion, peeled and chopped – 1
- Salt – ¾ teaspoon
- Ground black pepper – ½ teaspoon
- Almonds, chopped – ½ cup
- Cheddar cheese, grated – 1 pound
- Avocado mayonnaise – 2 cups

Directions:

1. Place all the ingredients for the dip in a medium bowl and stir until combined.
2. Divide dip evenly between small bowls and serve as a party dip.

Nutrition: calories: 184, fat: 12, fiber: 1, carbs: 4, protein: 5

Green Tabasco Devilled Eggs

Preparation Time: 20 minutes

Cooking Time: 10 minutes

Servings: 6

Ingredients:

- 6 Eggs
- 1/3 cup Mayonnaise
- 1 ½ tbsp. Green Tabasco
- Salt and Pepper, to taste

Directions:

1. Place the eggs in a saucepan over medium heat and pour boiling water over, enough to cover them.
2. Cook for 6-8 minutes.
3. Place in an ice bath to cool.
4. When safe to handle, peel the eggs and slice them in half.
5. Scoop out the yolks and place in a bowl.
6. Add the remaining ingredients.
7. Whisk to combine.

8. Fill the egg holes with the mixture.

9. Serve and enjoy!

Nutrition:

Calories 175

Total Fats 17g

Net Carbs: 5g

Protein 6g

Fiber: 1g

Herbed Cheese Balls

Preparation Time: 30 MIN

Cooking Time: 10 minutes

Servings: 20

Ingredients:

- 1/3 cup grated Parmesan Cheese
- 3 tbsp. Heavy Cream
- 4 tbsp. Butter, melted
- ¼ tsp Pepper
- 2 Eggs
- 1 cup Almond Flour
- ¼ cup Basil Leaves
- ¼ cup Parsley Leaves
- 2 tbsp. chopped Cilantro Leaves
- 1/3 cup crumbled Feta Cheese

Directions:

1. Place the ingredients in your food processor.
2. Pulse until the mixture becomes smooth.
3. Transfer to a bowl and freeze for 20 minutes or so, to set.
4. Shale the mixture into 20 balls.
5. Meanwhile, preheat the oven to 350 degrees F.
6. Arrange the cheese balls on a lined baking sheet.
7. Place in the oven and bake for 10 minutes.

8. Serve and enjoy!

Nutrition:

Calories 60 Total Fats 5g

Net Carbs: 8g Protein 2g

Fiber: 1g

Cheesy Salami Snack

Preparation Time: 30 MIN

Cooking Time: 10 minutes

Servings: 6

Ingredients:

- 4 ounces Cream Cheese
- 7 ounces dried Salami
- ¼ cup chopped Parsley

Directions:

1. Preheat the oven to 325 degrees F.
2. Slice the salami thinly (I got 30 slices).
3. Arrange the salami on a lined sheet and bake for 15 minutes.
4. Arrange on a serving platter and top each salami slice with a bit of cream cheese.
5. Serve and enjoy!

Nutrition:

Calories 139 Total Fats 15g

Net Carbs: 1g Protein 9g

Fiber: 0g

Pesto & Olive Fat Bombs

Preparation Time: 25 MIN

Cooking Time: 10 minutes

Servings: 8

Ingredients:

- 1 cup Cream Cheese
- 10 Olives, sliced

- 2 tbsp. Pesto Sauce
- ½ cup grated Parmesan Cheese

Directions:

1. Place all of the ingredients in a bowl.
2. Stir well to combine.
3. Place in the freezer and freeze for 15-20 minutes, to set.
4. Shape into 8 balls.
5. Serve and enjoy!

Nutrition:

Calories 123

Total Fats 13g

Net Carbs: 3g

Protein 4g

Fiber: 3g

Cheesy Broccoli Nuggets

Preparation Time: 25 MIN

Cooking Time: 10 minutes

Servings: 4

Ingredients:

- 1 cup shredded Cheese
- ¼ cup Almond Flour
- 2 cups Broccoli Florets, steamed in the microwave for 5 minutes
- 2 Egg Whites
- Salt and Pepper, to taste

Directions:

1. Preheat the oven to 350 degrees F.
2. Place the broccoli florets in a bowl and mash them with a potato masher.
3. Add the remaining ingredients and mix well with your hands, until combined.
4. Line a baking sheet with parchment paper.
5. Drop 20 scoops of the mixture onto the sheet.
6. Place in the oven and bake for 20 minutes or until golden.
7. Serve and enjoy!

Nutrition:

Calories 145

Total Fats 9g

Net Carbs: 4g

Protein 10g

Fiber: 1g

CHAPTER 12:

Desserts

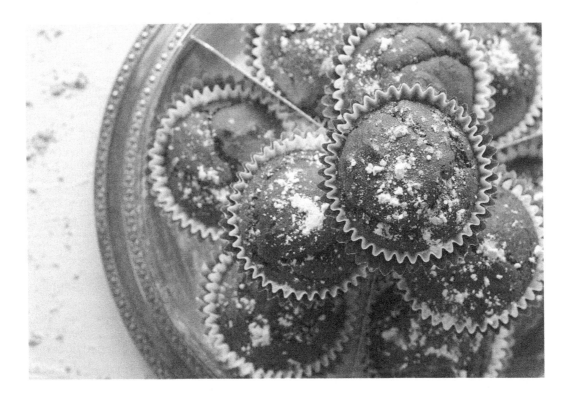

Southern Apple Pie

Preparation Time: 15 minutes

Cooking Time: 40 minutes

Servings: 8 persons

Ingredients

- Crust:
- 2 cups blanched almond flour
- ½ cup butter
- ½ cup powdered Erythritol
- 1 teaspoon allspice
- Filling:
- 3 cups sliced apples
- ¼ cup melted butter
- ½ lemon, juiced
- ¼ cup powdered Erythritol
- ½ teaspoon allspice
- Topping:
- Cinnamon, as desired
- Granulated Erythritol, as desired

Directions

1. Prepare the crust; preheat oven to 375F.
2. Melt the butter in a microwave safe bowl.
3. Combine almond flour, melted butter, and remaining crust ingredients until the dough comes together.
4. Press the crust into 9-inch springform.
5. Cover the crust with parchment paper and baking balls (or rice) and bake 10 minutes.
6. In the meantime, make the filling; toss the sliced apples with juice.
7. Remove the crust from the oven. Fill with the apples in a circular pattern.
8. Combine butter, Erythritol, and allspice in a bowl.
9. Pour over the apples.
10. Bake the pie for 30 minutes.
11. Remove the pie from the oven and allow to cool.
12. Combine desired amounts of cinnamon and Erythritol.
13. Sprinkle the apples with the cinnamon mixture.
14. Slice and serve.

Nutrition

Calories 123,

Fat 9.2g,

Carbs 4.8g,

Protein 8.3g

Cheese Berry Pie

Preparation Time: 15 minutes

Cooking Time: 25 minutes

Servings: 8 persons

Ingredients

- Crust:
- 1 cup coconut oil, solid
- 4 large eggs
- 1 pinch salt
- 1 ½ cups softened coconut flour
- 1 tablespoon cold water
- ½ teaspoon baking powder
- Filling:
- 1 ½ cups fresh blueberries
- 2 tablespoons granulated Erythritol
- 1 cup cream cheese

Directions

1. Preheat oven to350F.
2. Make the crust; combine coconut flour, salt, and baking powder in a bowl.
3. Work in coconut oil.

4. Add eggs, one at the time until incorporated.
5. Add water and stir until you have a smooth dough. Divide the dough into two equal parts.
6. Transfer the one part into 9-inch pie pan. Roll out the second and place aside.
7. Prepare the filling; spread cream cheese over the crust.
8. Toss the blueberries with the Erythritol and spread over the cheese.
9. Top the pie with the remaining dough.
10. Bake the pie for 25 minutes.
11. Cool the pie on a rack for 10 minutes.
12. Slice and serve.

Nutrition

Calories 143,

Fat 9.2g, Carbs 4.8g,

Protein 8.3g

Lemon Cheesecake

Preparation Time: 15 minutes

Cooking Time: 25 minutes

Servings: 12 persons

Ingredients

- Crust:
- 2 teaspoons granulated Erythritol
- 2 cups almond flour
- ½ cup unsalted melted butter
- ¼ cup desiccated coconut
- Filling:
- 1 tablespoon powdered gelatin
- 2 tablespoons granulated Erythritol
- ¾ cup boiling water
- ½ cup cold water
- 1lb. cream cheese
- 2 lemons, zested and juice

Directions

1. Prepare the crust; combine the crust ingredients in a large mixing bowl.
2. Stir until the dough comes together.
3. Transfer the dough into 9-inch springform.
4. Place in a fridge while you make the filling.
5. Prepare the filling; pour the water in a bowl. Sprinkle over the gelatin powder. Pour in cold water and place aside for 5 minutes.
6. Beat cream cheese, gelatin mixture, Erythritol, lemon juice and zest in a mixing bowl.
7. Pour the filling over the crust.
8. Refrigerate for 2 hours.
9. Slice and serve.

Nutrition

Calories 143,

Fat 9.2g, Carbs 4.8g,

Protein 8.3g

No-Guilt Chocolate Cake

Preparation Time: 15 minutes + inactive time

Cooking Time: 25 minutes

Servings: 8 persons

Ingredients

- ¾ cup butter
- 12oz. sugar-free quality dark chocolate, chopped or chocolate chips
- 1 teaspoon sugar-free vanilla extract
- 3 large eggs, room temperature
- 1 pinch salt
- ¼ cup granulated Erythritol
- 10 drops liquid Stevia

Directions

1. Preheat oven to 350F.
2. Line 8-inch springform pan with baking paper. Additionally, grease with some coconut oil for easy removal.
3. Melt butter and chopped chocolate over a double boiler.
4. Remove from the heat and pour the mixture into a large bowl.
5. Beat in vanilla and salt.
6. Beat in the eggs, one at the time, and beating well after each addition.
7. Fold in the sweetener.
8. Strain the mixture through a fine sieve into the prepared springform.
9. Gently tap the springform onto the kitchen counter.
10. Bake the cake for 25 minutes.
11. Cool the cake to room temperature and refrigerate for at least 8 hours.
12. Slice and serve, with a dollop of whipped coconut cream.

Nutrition

Calories 103,

Fat 9.2g, Carbs 4.8g,

Protein 8.3g

The Best Cookies

Preparation Time: 15 minutes

Cooking Time: 10 minutes

Servings: 16 persons

Ingredients

- 1/3 cup coconut oil
- 1 ½ teaspoon sugar-free vanilla extract
- 1 medium egg
- 1pinch salt
- 3 tablespoons granulated Erythritol
- 1 cup almond flour
- 2 tablespoons coconut flour
- ½ teaspoon cinnamon
- 1/3 cup sugar-free quality dark chocolate chips

Directions

1. Preheat oven to 350F. Line baking sheet with a parchment paper.
2. In a mixing bowl, beat egg with vanilla and Erythritol.
3. Melt the coconut oil and fold into the egg mixture.
4. Fold in the remaining ingredients and stir until the dough comes together.
5. Let the dough stand for 5 minutes.
6. Scoop the dough with a cookie scoop, onto the baking sheet.
7. Press gently with the back of your spoon to flatten.
8. Bake the cookies for 10 minutes.
9. Cool briefly on a wire rack before serving.
10. Serve with a cup of almond milk and enjoy.

Nutrition

Calories 143,

Fat 9.2g, Carbs 4.8g,

Protein 8.3

Salty Caramel Cake

Preparation Time: 15 minutes

Cooking Time: 25 minutes

Servings: 10 persons

Ingredients

- 2 cups blanched almond flour
- 3 tablespoons coconut flour
- 2 tablespoons vanilla whey protein powder
- ¾ tablespoon baking powder

- 1/3 cup unsalted butter
- 1 pinch salt
- ½ cup granulated Erythritol
- 3 large eggs, room temperature
- 1 teaspoon sugar-free vanilla extract
- ½ cup unsweetened almond milk
- 2 cups sugar-free caramel sauce
- Sea salt flakes, for sprinkle

Directions

1. Preheat oven to 325F.
2. Line 2 8-inch spring form pans with baking paper.
3. In a mixing bowl, combine all the dry ingredients, except the sweetener.
4. In a separate bowl, cream butter, and Erythritol.
5. Beat in eggs, one at the time, followed by vanilla and almond milk
6. Fold the liquid ingredients into the dry ones.
7. Divide the batter between two spring form pans.
8. Bake the sponges for 25 minutes or until the inserted toothpick comes out clean.
9. Place the sponges aside to cool.
10. Spread 1 ½ cups of the caramel sauce over one sponge. Top with the second sponge.
11. Pour the remaining caramel over the top.
12. Sprinkle the caramel with salt flakes. Refrigerate the cake for 1 hour. Slice and serve.

Nutrition

Calories 143,

Fat 9.2g, Carbs 4.8g,

Protein 8.3g

Luscious Red Velvet Cake

Preparation Time: 15 minutes + inactive time

Cooking Time: 25 minutes

Servings: 10 persons

Ingredients

- Cake:
- 1 cup granulated Erythritol
- ½ cup coconut flour
- ½ cup Swerve
- 2 tablespoons raw cocoa powder
- 6 large eggs, separated
- ½ cup melted and cooled butter
- 2 tablespoons crème Fraiche
- 1 tablespoon powdered red food coloring
- 1 teaspoon white vinegar
- 1 teaspoon sugar-free vanilla
- Frosting:
- 4oz. cream cheese
- 4 tablespoons softened unsalted butter
- 2 cups Swerve
- 1 tablespoon heavy cream
- ½ teaspoon sugar-free vanilla extract

Directions

1. Preheat oven to 350F.
2. Line 9-inch springform with a baking paper and grease with some coconut oil.
3. Combine all the dry ingredients in a large mixing bowl.
4. In a separate bowl, beat eggs, butter, crème Fraiche, vinegar, and vanilla.
5. Fold the liquid ingredients into the dry ones and stir until smooth.
6. Pour the batter into the springform.

7. Bake the cake for 25-30 minutes or until the inserted toothpick comes out clean.
8. Make the frosting; beat cream cheese and butter in a bowl until fluffy.
9. Add sugar and heavy cream.
10. Beat until smooth.
11. Remove the cake from the springform once completely cold.
12. Top with the frosting.
13. Refrigerate the cake for 30 minutes.
14. Slice and serve.

Nutrition

Calories 143,

Fat 9.2g, Carbs 4.8g,

Protein 8.3g

Southern Pecan Pie

Preparation Time: 15 minutes

Cooking Time: 50 minutes

Servings: 10 persons

Ingredients

- Crust:
- 3 cups blanched almond flour
- 4 large eggs, room temperature
- ½ cup unsalted melted butter
- ½ cup Swerve
- 1 good pinch salt
- Filling:
- 1 cup coconut oil or butter
- ¾ cup golden Swerve
- ½ cup granulated Erythritol
- 1 ½ tablespoon sugar-free maple syrup
- 4 large eggs, room temperature
- 1 ½ cup pecans, chopped
- ¾ cup pecan halves
- 2 teaspoon vanilla-bourbon extract

Directions

1. Preheat oven to 325F.
2. Grease 10-inch cast iron skillet with butter.
3. In a large mixing bowl, combine the crust ingredients until the smooth dough is formed.
4. Transfer the dough into the skillet and press so you cover the bottom and sides.
5. Prepare the filling; melt butter in a saucepot and fold in sweeteners and sugar-free maple syrup. Stir until the sweeteners are dissolved. Place aside to cool.
6. Beat the eggs with cold syrup until fluffy. Fold in pecan pieces.
7. Pour the sauce into the crust.
8. Top with pecan halves.
9. Cover the pie with an aluminum foil. Bake the pie for 40 minutes.
10. Cool before slicing and serving.

Nutrition

Calories 143,

Fat 9.2g, Carbs 4.8g,

Protein 8.3g

Roasted Brussels sprouts With Pecans and Gorgonzola

Preparation Time: 10 minutes

Cooking Time: 35 minutes

Servings: 4

Ingredients:

- Brussels Sprouts, fresh- 1 pound
- Pecans, chopped- ¼ cup
- Olive oil- 1 tablespoon
- Extra olive oil to oil the baking tray
- Pepper and salt for tasting

- Gorgonzola cheese- ¼ cup (If you prefer not to use the Gorgonzola cheese, you can toss the Brussels sprouts when hot, with 2 tablespoons of butter instead.

Directions:

1. Warm the oven to 350 degrees Fahrenheit or 175 Celsius.
2. Rub a large pan or any vessel you wish to use with a little bit of olive oil. You can use a paper towel or a pastry brush.
3. Cut off the ends of the Brussels sprouts if you need to and then cut then in a lengthwise direction into halves. (Fear not if a few of the leaves come off of them, some may become deliciously crunchy during cooking)
4. Chop up all of the pecans using a knife and then measure them for the amount.
5. Put your Brussels sprouts as well as the sliced pecans inside a bowl, and cover them all with some olive oil, pepper, and salt (be generous).
6. Arrange all of your pecans and Brussels sprouts onto your roasting pan in a single layer
7. Roast this for 30 to 35 minutes, or when they become tender and can be pierced with a fork easily. Stir during cooking if you wish to get a more even browning.
8. Once cooked, toss them with the Gorgonzola Cheese (or butter) before you serve them. Serve them hot.

Nutrition:

Calories: 149, Fat: 11 grams,

Carbohydrates: 10 grams,

Fiber: 4 grams,

Protein: 5 grams

Almond Flour Muffins

Preparation Time: 15 minutes

Cooking Time: 30 minutes

Servings: 8

Ingredients:

- 1/3 cup of pumpkin puree
- 3 eggs
- 2 tablespoons agave nectar
- 2 tablespoons coconut oil
- 1 teaspoon vanilla extract
- 1 teaspoon white vinegar
- 1 cup chopped fruits
- 1 teaspoon baking soda
- ½ teaspoon salt

Directions:

1. Preheat the oven to 350°F.
2. Line the muffin tin with paper liners
3. In the first mixing bowl, whisk the almond flour, salt, and baking soda.
4. In the second mixing bowl, whisk the pumpkin puree, eggs, coconut oil, agave nectar, vanilla extract, and vinegar.
5. Now add this puree mix of the second bowl to the first bowl and blend everything well.
6. Add the chopped fruits to the blend.
7. Pour the mixture to the muffin cups in your pan.
8. Bake for 15-20 minutes. Ensure that the contents have set in the center, and a golden brown lining has started to appear at the edges.
9. Transfer the muffins to a cooling rack and let it cool completely.

Nutrition:

Calories: 75, Carbs: 4 grams,

Fat: 6 grams, Protein: 0 gram

Chocolate Ganache

Preparation Time: 10 minutes

Cooking Time: 16 minutes

Servings: 16

Size/ Portion: 2 tablespoons

Ingredients

- 9 ounces bittersweet chocolate, chopped
- 1 cup heavy cream
- 1 tablespoon dark rum (optional)

Direction

1. Situate chocolate in a medium bowl. Cook cream in a small saucepan over medium heat.
2. Bring to a boil. When the cream has reached a boiling point, pour the chopped chocolate over it and beat until smooth. Stir the rum if desired.
3. Allow the ganache to cool slightly before you pour it on a cake. Begin in the middle of the cake and work outside. For a fluffy icing or chocolate filling, let it cool until thick and beat with a whisk until light and fluffy.

Nutrition:

142 calories 10.8g fat 1.4g protein

Chocolate Covered Strawberries

Preparation Time: 15 minutes

Cooking Time: 0 minute

Servings: 24

Size/ Portion: 2 pieces

Ingredients

- 16 ounces milk chocolate chips
- 2 tablespoons shortening
- 1-pound fresh strawberries with leaves

Direction

1. In a bain-marie, melt chocolate and shortening, occasionally stirring until smooth. Pierce the tops of the strawberries with toothpicks and immerse them in the chocolate mixture.
2. Turn the strawberries and put the toothpick in Styrofoam so that the chocolate cools.

Nutrition:

115 calories

7.3g fat

1.4g protein

Strawberry Angel Food Dessert

Difficulty: Novice level

Preparation Time: 15 minutes

Cooking Time: 0 minutes

Servings: 18

Size/ Portion: 1 cup

Ingredients

- 1 angel cake (10 inches)
- 2 packages of softened cream cheese
- 1 cup of white sugar
- 1 container (8 oz.) of frozen fluff, thawed
- 1 liter of fresh strawberries, sliced
- 1 jar of strawberry icing

Direction

1. Crumble the cake in a 9 x 13-inch dish.
2. Beat the cream cheese and sugar in a medium bowl until the mixture is light and fluffy. Stir in the whipped topping. Crush the cake with your

hands, and spread the cream cheese mixture over the cake.

3. Combine the strawberries and the frosting in a bowl until the strawberries are well covered. Spread over the layer of cream cheese. Cool until ready to serve.

Nutrition:

261 calories

11g fat

3.2g protein

Rhubarb Strawberry Crunch

Preparation Time: 15 minutes

Cooking Time: 45 minutes

Servings: 18

Size/ Portion: 1 cup

Ingredients

- 1 cup of white sugar
- 3 tablespoons all-purpose flour
- 3 cups of fresh strawberries, sliced
- 3 cups of rhubarb, cut into cubes
- 1 1/2 cup flour
- 1 cup packed brown sugar
- 1 cup butter
- 1 cup oatmeal

Direction

1. Preheat the oven to 190 ° C.
2. Combine white sugar, 3 tablespoons flour, strawberries and rhubarb in a large bowl. Place the mixture in a 9 x 13-inch baking dish.
3. Mix 1 1/2 cups of flour, brown sugar, butter, and oats until a crumbly texture is obtained. You may want to use a blender for this. Crumble the mixture of rhubarb and strawberry.

4. Bake for 45 minutes.

Nutrition:

253 calories 10.8g fat 2.3g protein

Chocolate Chip Banana Dessert

Preparation Time: 20 minutes

Cooking Time: 20 minutes

Servings: 24

Size/ Portion:

Ingredients

- 2/3 cup white sugar
- 3/4 cup butter
- 2/3 cup brown sugar
- 1 egg, beaten slightly
- 1 teaspoon vanilla extract
- 1 cup of banana puree
- 1 3/4 cup flour
- 2 teaspoons baking powder
- 1/2 teaspoon of salt
- 1 cup of semi-sweet chocolate chips

Direction:

1. Ready the oven to 175 ° C Grease and bake a 10 x 15-inch baking pan.
2. Beat the butter, white sugar, and brown sugar in a large bowl until light. Beat the egg and vanilla. Fold in the banana puree: mix baking powder, flour, and salt in another bowl. Mix flour mixture into the butter mixture. Stir in the chocolate chips. Spread in pan.
3. Bake for 20 minutes. Cool before cutting into squares.

Nutrition:

174 calories 8.2g fat 1.7g protein

Apple Pie Filling

Preparation Time: 20 minutes

Cooking Time: 12 minutes

Servings: 40

Size/ Portion: 1 cup

Ingredients

- 18 cups chopped apples
- 3 tablespoons lemon juice
- 10 cups of water
- 4 1/2 cups of white sugar
- 1 cup corn flour
- 2 teaspoons of ground cinnamon
- 1 teaspoon of salt
- 1/4 teaspoon ground nutmeg

Direction

1. Mix apples with lemon juice in a large bowl and set aside. Pour the water in a Dutch oven over medium heat. Combine sugar, corn flour, cinnamon, salt, and nutmeg in a bowl. Add to water, mix well, and bring to a boil. Cook for 2 minutes with continuous stirring.
2. Boil apples again. Reduce the heat, cover, and simmer for 8 minutes. Allow cooling for 30 minutes.
3. Pour into five freezer containers and leave 1/2 inch of free space. Cool to room temperature.
4. Seal and freeze

Nutrition:

129 calories

0.1g fat

0.2g protein

Ice Cream Sandwich Dessert

Preparation Time: 20 minutes

Cooking Time: 0 minute

Servings: 12

Size/ Portion: 2 squares

Ingredients

- 22 ice cream sandwiches
- Frozen whipped topping in 16 oz. container, thawed
- 1 jar (12 oz.) Caramel ice cream
- 1 1/2 cups of salted peanuts

Direction

1. Cut a sandwich with ice in two. Place a whole sandwich and a half sandwich on a short side of a 9 x 13-inch baking dish. Repeat this until the bottom is covered, alternate the full sandwich, and the half sandwich.
2. Spread half of the whipped topping. Pour the caramel over it. Sprinkle with half the peanuts. Do layers with the rest of the ice cream sandwiches, whipped cream, and peanuts.
3. Cover and freeze for up to 2 months. Remove from the freezer 20 minutes before serving. Cut into squares.

Nutrition:

559 calories 28.8g fat10g protein

Cranberry and Pistachio Biscotti

Preparation Time: 15 minutes

Cooking Time: 35 minutes

Servings: 36

Size/ Portion: 2 slices

Ingredients

- 1/4 cup light olive oil
- 3/4 cup white sugar

- 2 teaspoons vanilla extract
- 1/2 teaspoon almond extract
- 2 eggs
- 1 3/4 cup all-purpose flour
- 1/4 teaspoon salt
- 1 teaspoon baking powder
- 1/2 cup dried cranberries
- 1 1/2 cup pistachio nuts

Direction

1. Prep oven to 150 ° C
2. Combine the oil and sugar in a large bowl until a homogeneous mixture is obtained. Stir in the vanilla and almond extract and add the eggs. Combine flour, salt, and baking powder; gradually add to the egg mixture — mix cranberries and nuts by hand.
3. Divide the dough in half — form two 12 x 2-inch logs on a parchment baking sheet. The dough can be sticky, wet hands with cold water to make it easier to handle it.
4. Bake in the preheated oven for 35 minutes or until the blocks are golden brown. Pullout from the oven and let cool for 10 minutes. Reduce oven heat to 275 degrees F (135 degrees C).
5. Cut diagonally into 3/4-inch-thick slices. Place on the sides on the baking sheet covered with parchment — Bake for about 8 to 10 minutes

Nutrition:

92 calories

4.3g fat

2.1g protein

Cream Puff Dessert

Preparation Time: 20 minutes

Cooking Time: 36 minutes

Servings: 12

Size/ Portion: 2 puffs

Ingredients

Puff

- 1 cup water
- 1/2 cup butter
- 1 cup all-purpose flour
- 4 eggs

Filling

- 1 (8-oz) package cream cheese, softened
- 3 1/2 cups cold milk
- 2 (4-oz) packages instant chocolate pudding mix

Topping

- 1 (8-oz) package frozen whipped cream topping, thawed
- 1/4 cup topping with milk chocolate flavor
- 1/4 cup caramel filling
- 1/3 cup almond flakes

Direction:

1. Set oven to 200 degrees C (400 degrees F). Grease a 9 x 13-inch baking dish.
2. Melt the butter in the water in a medium-sized pan over medium heat. Pour the flour in one go and mix vigorously until the mixture forms a ball. Remove from heat and let stand for 5 minutes. Beat the eggs one by one until they are smooth and shiny. Spread in the prepared pan.

3. Bake in the preheated oven for 30 to 35 minutes, until puffed and browned. Cool completely on a rack.

4. While the puff pastry cools, mix the cream cheese mixture, the milk, and the pudding. Spread over the cooled puff pastry. Cool for 20 minutes.

5. Spread whipped cream on cooled topping and sprinkle with chocolate and caramel sauce. Sprinkle with almonds. Freeze 1 hour before serving.

Nutrition:

355 calories

22.3g fat

8.7g protein

Conclusion

Thanks for downloading this book. In this book, you were provided a variety of keto-friendly recipes. From cooking keto-friendly breakfast, lunch, and dinner, to fun different takes on snacking and yummy desserts, this book offers all the variety for a healthy, well-rounded diet plan. Be sure to keep the diet plan and the keto-shopping list nearby to make things easier. The recipes in this book are not just simple to understand but will help you whip up delicious and nutritious meals in no time.

With Ketogenic diet, you have to avoid or limit your consumption of carbs to less than 5% of your daily dietary intake. Secondly, you need to avoid unhealthy carbs such as tubers, starches, sugar, and other foods.

Once you have all of the chief spices and other fixings stocked in your keto kitchen, the following week's shopping list will be much simpler. As a quick reminder, keep these simple tips in mind as you go through your ketogenic journey:

Drink plenty of water daily and limit the intake of sugar-sweetened beverages.

It is essential to attempt to use only half of your typical serving of salad dressing or butter.

Use only fat-free or low-fat condiments.

Add a serving of vegetables to your dinner and lunch menus.

Add a serving of fruit as a snack or enjoy with your meal. The skin also contains additional nutrients. Dried and canned fruits are quick and easy to use. However, make sure they don't have added sugar.

Read the food labels and make choices that keep you in line with ketosis.

A snack has some frozen yogurt (fat-free or low-fat), nuts or unsalted pretzels, raw veggies, and unsalted-plain popcorn.

Prepare cut veggies such as bell pepper strips, mixed greens, and carrots. Store them in small baggies for a quick on-the-go healthy choice.

One of the easiest ways to stay on your plan is to remove the temptations. Remove the chocolate, candy, bread, pasta, rice, and sugary sodas you have supplied in your kitchen. If you live alone, this is an easy task. It is a bit more challenging if you have a family. The diet will also be useful for them if you plan your meals using the recipes included in this book.

If you cheat, that has to count also. It will be a reminder of your indulgence, but it will help keep you in line. Others may believe you are obsessed with the plan, but it is your health and wellbeing that you are improving.

When you go shopping for your ketogenic essentials be sure you take your new skills, a grocery list, and search the labels. Almost every food item in today's grocery store has a nutrition label. Be sure you read each ingredient to discover any hiding carbs to keep your ketosis in line. You will be glad you took the extra time.

Made in the USA
Monee, IL
30 March 2021